M000043594

Advance Praise for ***The Glutened Human***

As someone who's been gluten free for 7 years, wow I'm learning so much that I didn't know! I LOVE this book! Dr. Shikhman has a way of answering all the questions you have, including the questions you didn't know you had. I couldn't put it down. Every time I turned a page, it helped me understand celiac disease and gluten intolerance a little more, even after all these years. Trust me, no matter if you are seeking answers and wondering if you are gluten intolerant, or if you have celiac disease and have been gluten free for 20 years, you want to read this book. It's a goldmine of knowledge that should be on everyone's shelf, for us, for our kids and for every person who's yet to be diagnosed. Thank you, Dr. Shikhman, for writing this book. It gives me chills knowing how many people will be helped, and spared years of pain, because of the light bulb moments that will happen through experiencing this book. Amazing.

Lauren Lucille Vasser
"The Celiac Diva"

Knowledge is power and in his book *The Glutened Human*, Dr. Shikhman gives us the power to heal. The book is thoughtfully laid out to educate about Celiac Disease and Gluten Intolerance and the many possible associated health issues and does so in a manner that is understandable. More importantly, Dr. Shikhman provides solutions and lifestyle modifications to combat those issues. Interspersed are real life stories from people who have suffered - and recovered - from the myriad of symptoms and conditions stemming from gluten. These stories prove to us that we are not alone and offer hope. With *The Glutened Human*, Dr. Shikhman provides us with knowledge that empowers us to take control of our physical well-being and leads us on the path to better health.

Carol Kicinski
Founder & Editor-in-Chief
Simply Gluten Free

The Glutened Human

Real stories from a medical practice and the science of how gluten causes ailments varying from chronic pain and autoimmune diseases to metabolic and psychiatric illnesses

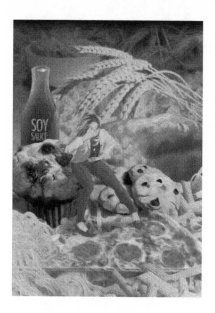

By

Dr. Alexander Shikhman MD, PhD

With

Dr. David Lemberg

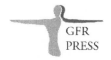

GFR
PRESS

DR. ALEXANDER SHIKHMAN / DR. DAVID LEMBERG

GFR Press
San Diego, CA
www.glutenfreeremedies.com

© 2016 Dr. Alexander Shikhman MD, PhD. All Rights Reserved,

No part of this book may be reproduced, stored in a retrieval system, or
transmitted by any means without the written permission of the author.

ISBN 10: 0692640223 (sc)
ISBN 13: 978-0692640227 (sc)
Printed in the United States of America
North Charleston, South Carolina

This book is printed on acid-free paper made from 30% post-consumer waste recycled material.

Library of Congress Control Number: 2016902677
GFR Press, San Diego CA

Book Cover and Page Design: Matthew J. Pallamary/San Diego CA
Cover Art: Marshall Ross/San Diego CA
Author's Photographs: Mark Dasktrup/San Diego CA

AUTHOR'S NOTE

THE GLUTENED HUMAN...

My professional journey into the world of food as a trigger of human illnesses started in the late 90s when I began practicing rheumatology at Scripps Clinic in La Jolla, CA.

Most of my day was spent at The Scripps Research Institute, and my long evening hours were dedicated to patient care in the clinic. During one of the evenings, I consulted a patient with debilitating psoriasis and psoriatic arthritis. He could barely walk, and his skin, including his face and hands, were completely covered with active psoriatic lesions. The unusualness of the consultation was due to his religious beliefs; he declined my offers of traditional medical therapy and requested a "natural" approach to his illness. I was confused and frustrated. I did not have enough expertise in the area of "natural" therapy of autoimmune diseases, but as a professional I wanted to help the patient and respect his requests. The next several days I spent in the library trying to find any relevant information on natural therapies for his condition. The information was very limited and not very impressive.

Incidentally, I came across patient testimonials that showed companies in Europe performing food intolerance testing had success with food elimination protocols in psoriasis and psoriatic arthritis. I gave my patient this information and wished him luck. I was very skeptical that such an approach would make a difference, but to my surprise, he showed up several months later with nearly normal skin and his joint pain was not bothering him at all. With a great smile on his face, he informed me that the food intolerance testing performed in the UK revealed that he was strongly intolerant to salmon, which he was eating almost every day. Elimination of the salmon from his diet resulted in a dramatic improvement of his health, and more importantly, the effect of the diet was long lasting.

Being intrigued by the patient's success, I started analyzing the effect of diet on patient health, and soon realized that compared to other products, gluten containing foods had a major negative impact on autoimmune and metabolic ailments. Since this discovery, a gluten-free diet has become a vital part of my therapeutic protocols. I became familiar with the term "glutened" after my patients, who were on a gluten free diet, accidentally ate gluten and became sick. Now the term "glutened" is widely accepted to mean negative symptoms due to gluten exposure. *The Glutened Human* shares successful stories of patients cured by a gluten-free diet and discusses the actual scientific data explaining their success.

In 2008, I founded Institute for Specialized Medicine, a clinic of integrative rheumatology, a place where we help patients not only by treating their symptoms, but also by unveiling the potential driving forces behind their illness. While scientifically based, our integrative approach relies heavily on the rational use of Western medicine combined with dietary interventions, food supplements and herbs as well as various physical therapeutic factors such as physical therapy, pilates, light therapy, and kinesiology among others.

In search for food supplements better suitable for the problems we treat in our clinic, in 2011 we introduced Gluten-Free Remedies, a line of professional, gluten-free-certified food supplements. Our supplements have helped our patients and customers across the country find a safe, effective alternative to many traditional drugs.

Enjoy the book and remember: it is never too late...

Dr. Alexander Shikhman MD, PhD

INTRODUCTION

The Greek physician Hippocrates said, "Let food be thy medicine and medicine be thy food." Indeed, what we eat is the cornerstone to our physical well-being, yet sometimes what we *don't* eat can save our lives.

My Story

My life has always been full of adventure. After graduating from college, I lived on three different continents and traveled the world visiting more than thirty countries. I tried everything from sailing in New Zealand while completing my Master's Degree, to working as one of the first Peace Corps Volunteers in a tiny Zambian village eating fried caterpillars and building wells and latrines near a crocodile-infested river. I had success as a scientific and technical writer. I skydived, bungee jumped, and ran marathons to raise money for charities. I had a zest for living and nothing slowed me down. Then at age 32, I collapsed in the shower and was rushed to the hospital where I started fighting for my life. I inexplicably developed more than twenty-six symptoms including: excruciating neck pain, dizziness, exhaustion, abdominal pain, severe muscle weakness, neurological symptoms, and a rapid heartbeat. The physicians were baffled. My independence was ripped away, causing the loss of my job, financial security, many friends, and any semblance of the life I once knew.

My persistent malady led to years of suffering, during which time my condition worsened to the point of having 911 on speed dial. I was told I had chronic fatigue and fibromyalgia, but that didn't explain many of my symptoms. I tried anything and everything— from outlandish treatments to eccentric healers. Nothing helped. I felt lost, alone, and afraid. The longer I went undiagnosed, the more doctors, friends, and family members questioned my sanity. Over time, I began questioning it too. One doctor told me, "It's all in your head." Another said, "You just need some anti-depressants."

Eventually my body reacted to almost every food I ate with hives, burning sensations, neuropathy, stomach distention, and diarrhea. Bedridden, emaciated, and spoon fed to stay alive, I had almost given up hope that I could ever be helped. Hospitalized yet again for traumatic symptoms without answers, an emergency room doctor scribbled a name of a rheumatologist, placed the paper in my hand and said, "Go see him. If anyone can help you, he can."
Two weeks later I had an appointment to see this rheumatologist, Dr. Alexander Shikhman, at his clinic, Institute for Specialized Medicine. He told me I wasn't going to make it much longer. After years of suffering, my body was shutting down. He conducted a battery of tests and put me on steroids to keep me alive while we waited for the results.

The answers were alarming. He explained I suffered from a variety of ailments, including Sjogrens syndrome (an autoimmune disease), leaky gut syndrome, and severe iron and vitamin deficiencies, all complicated by gluten intolerance. He started me on a series of treatments, including a strict gluten-free diet, and supplements to treat the damage to my immune system and gut from the years of being ill and eating gluten. He was caring and listened; and it felt wonderful to be heard by someone with the right knowledge to help me.

By following Dr. Shikhman's instructions, I began to feel substantially better within months. I had been told by other health care practitioners, years prior, that it would be helpful to avoid eating gluten and sugar because I had been diagnosed with candidiasis (an overgrowth of yeast in the body). I was never strict about it until I met Dr. Shikhman, who explained the damage gluten, even in the slightest amount, caused to my digestive and immune system. I haven't eaten gluten since.

Now six years later, I am still on a strict diet, completely free of gluten, dairy, soy, sugar, and other food allergens particular to my needs. I went from the precipice of death to living again. I feel grateful to have survived and I owe much of that to Dr. Shikhman. Indeed, what you *don't* eat may very well save your life.

Often when it comes to our health, we can feel powerless. Since the advent of the Internet, this has been less true. A vast wealth of information is at our fingertips. With the myriad of information available to us, we can often become overwhelmed, lost, and confused. In *The Glutened Human*, Dr. Shikhman has built a bridge that will help you understand the connection that gluten intolerance and celiac disease may have with your health. The core message is that you are not alone and you can heal.

Believe you are superior to your circumstances. Empower yourself. Read this book and start your path to optimal health.

Wishing you the best of health and happiness,

–Cherie Kephart, M.A., author of *A Few Minor Adjustments*

TABLE OF CONTENTS

1   *Homo glutenicus*   15

2   Gluten and Autoimmune Disease   29

     Gluten Intolerance Self-Assessment   46

3   Gluten Intolerance and Psychiatric Disorders:
     Autism, Schizophrenia, and ADHD   48

4   Gluten Intolerance and Endocrine Disorders:
     Diabetes, Thyroid Disease, and Addison's Disease   67

5   The Cancer Connection   83

6   The Science of Gluten Intolerance and Celiac Disease   97

7   Leaky Gut Syndrome   119

     Leaky Gut Syndrome Self-Assessment   129

8   Disorders of Pregnancy, Infertility, and Osteoporosis
     Associated with Gluten Intolerance and Celiac Disease   141

9   Probiotics and Prebiotics   153

10   The Way Forward   170

11   Practicing the Gluten Free Lifestyle   186

12   Beyond Gluten Free: When a Gluten Free Diet Isn't Enough   213

     Yeast Infection (Candidiasis) Self-Assessment   217

13   Basic Lifestyle Modifications When Living With Gluten
     Intolerance, Celiac Disease, and Related Conditions   224

14   In Conclusion   233

     Gluten-Free Remedies: Natural Secrets to Better Health   238

     Bibliography   265

Homo glutenicus

One Woman's Story

Melanie Turner was a healthy, dynamic young woman in 1992 at age 18 when she went away to college. She had been an active child, teenager, and co-captain of her high school lacrosse team until her first year of college when numerous medical problems surfaced. After only a few months of freshman dormitory living, she began to experience severe numbness in her hands and feet. At times, "the numbness was so intense I couldn't feel my legs and feet when I was walking." Soon, the numbness ascended her legs all the way up to her knees.

Melanie's family physician referred her to a rheumatologist who diagnosed her with Raynaud's disease, a disorder caused by spasm of the arteries in the arms and legs. Her doctor prescribed Procardia, a calcium channel blocker frequently used to treat angina, (chest pain caused by a lack of sufficient oxygen reaching the heart muscle). Procardia works by relaxing the smooth muscle contained in arterial walls and is often used to treat Raynaud's disease, but Melanie didn't respond well to the drug. "I didn't feel right," she said, "and my heart bothered me."

Additionally, Melanie suffered from extreme abdominal pain, which was diagnosed as an "intestinal infection." She became "sick all the time" and battled frequent yeast and bladder infections. A number of doctors prescribed various antibiotics, and over the course of many months, Melanie was given penicillin, amoxicillin, Cipro, and others. Ultimately, blood tests showed that her liver enzymes were elevated and Melanie was diagnosed with autoimmune hepatitis. An endocrinologist prescribed prednisone for treatment of the autoimmune liver disease.

Melanie continued having "one problem after another." Severe and persistent joint pains soon made her situation worse. Joint pain is often associated with autoimmune hepatitis, therefore, another drug–sulindac–was added to the growing list of Melanie's daily medications, but she developed severe side effects from the drug, including fever and a widespread rash, so sulindac was withdrawn.

During the next few years, Melanie developed muscle weakness, persistent fatigue and was diagnosed with Hashimoto's thyroiditis, another autoimmune disorder. Accordingly, she was placed on a regimen of thyroid hormone replacement therapy (Synthroid).

In her early 20s, Melanie endured several bouts of pleurisy, an inflammation of the membranes surrounding the lungs. She also developed ulcers of the mucous membranes of her mouth and a skin disorder known as dermatitis herpetiformis.

Melanie continued taking prednisone for her liver condition and developed many food allergies throughout her 20s, saying "I got to the point where I was allergic to more foods than the ones I could eat." She also became allergic to the most commonly prescribed antibiotics and continued to suffer frequent yeast and urinary tract infections.

At 27 years old, a rheumatologist told Melanie she had lupus (systemic lupus erythematosusm SLE). Melanie had experienced all of the disturbing symptoms of lupus including fatigue, hair loss, pleurisy, joint pains, and mouth ulcers as well as periodic worsening of symptoms known as "flares." In 2001 she had a serious flare and developed pericarditis, a dangerous condition involving an accumulation of fluid around the heart.

In spite of everything, Melanie got married, and at age 32 became pregnant, but following successful delivery of her baby girl, Melanie's gastrointestinal pain and constipation worsened. Once again, she found herself sitting in a doctor's office, but this time an astute gastroenterologist finally identified the diagnosis that explained almost all of Melanie's problems: celiac disease. The doctor recommended a gluten-free diet. Celiac disease and its precursor, gluten intolerance could account for the majority of Melanie's extensive list of health problems.

Gluten intolerance and celiac disease are terms that describe a continuum of signs and symptoms involving an immunologic response and inflammatory reaction to gluten. Gluten proteins are contained in wheat, barley, and rye, staple grains of the Western diet and is abundant in breads, flours, pastries, pizza, pasta, breakfast cereals, gravies, sauces, and soups. Almost 40% of Americans and Western Europeans are genetically susceptible to gluten intolerance. A proportion of these individuals, like Melanie, can develop immune reactions to gluten, which can result in a wide variety of diseases.

Genetic susceptibility as well as various environmental triggers can cause certain individuals to develop signs and symptoms of gluten intolerance which can be considered early stages of an immunologic response to gluten. Celiac disease is as an autoimmune disease where eating gluten causes damage to the small intestine. It is a multisystem disorder which can involve the gastrointestinal, immune, endocrine, reproductive, muscle, and nerve systems.

Melanie attempted to follow a gluten free program, eliminating products containing wheat, rye, and barley. She had recently given birth and felt a need to add protein to her diet, so she began drinking a protein-rich, rice-based liquid thinking it would be safe, as rice contains no gluten, but after a few days Melanie's gastrointestinal symptoms, including persistent diarrhea and abdominal pain, increased, and she began to lose weight. At 5 feet 4 inches tall, she became markedly underweight, weighing only 90 pounds. She returned to the most recent physician who had diagnosed her with celiac disease, and he explained that the protein drink contained wheat-based fillers and was a significant source of "hidden" gluten. (Unfortunately, many manufactured foods that do not list wheat, barley, or rye among their ingredients still contain trace amounts of gluten, and such a concentration may be enough to provoke a serious reaction in a gluten-intolerant person.)

In the spring of 2006, Melanie began a new gluten free food plan with high hopes. The dramatic results were gratifying and immediate. Melanie regained 15 pounds within a few months, was living pain-free, and no longer experienced the debilitating diarrhea caused by hidden gluten in the rice drink.

Within two years, Melanie experienced even more remarkable

benefits of being gluten-free. Her allergies to a long list of foods receded and the spring and fall seasonal allergies she had endured for more than 10 years decreased in intensity, indicated by less itching, sneezing, and mucous membrane irritation. Additionally, her autoimmune hepatitis stabilized and her liver enzymes fell to lower levels allowing her to reduce her daily dosage of prednisone.

"I recovered a lot," Melanie said. Her gluten free food plan was working and many of her illnesses had largely resolved or, like the autoimmune hepatitis, had stabilized. Her joint pain subsided, but she continued to experience chronic fatigue, possibly related to lupus, as well as nerve pain in her hands and feet, related to Raynaud's disease. Her hair was also very thin, but even with these residual symptoms, her overall health was much improved.

In 2007 Melanie felt a pain in her right hip and fell down. An x-ray showed avascular necrosis in both hips. In avascular necrosis, the blood supply to a region of bone is interrupted and the affected bone begins to die. If avascular necrosis involves a joint such as the hip, both the surrounding bone and the joint cartilage may be affected. Melanie's ability to walk normally was in jeopardy.

She wanted to find a doctor who could "put all the pieces together," and treated her for one major condition rather than individual unrelated treatments for "ten different diagnoses." She made some calls and was recommended to our clinic, the Institute for Specialized Medicine, a center for integrative rheumatology in San Diego, California. After a physical examination and review of laboratory tests, we confirmed Melanie's earlier diagnosis of celiac disease, as well as immune reactions to dairy and egg proteins. We took her off prednisone and substituted prednisolone, another steroid that prevents the release of substances in the body that cause inflammation, enabling her body to do much less work. We also instructed her to eliminate dairy and eggs from her diet.

Melanie followed our advice and within two months her hair grew back, and she had "way more energy." She now walks regularly for exercise and began jogging "for the first time in two-and-a-half years". She is now 43 and the mother of a 10-year old daughter. She says, "I am so much better than I was 10 years ago." The key actions that made the difference were a completely gluten-free diet and eliminating dairy products and eggs, which were identified as additional immune system triggers.

Melanie describes herself as being very healthy when she was growing up. What happened to her? Now, Melanie is able to clearly identify the turning point. When she was a child her mother did all the cooking from scratch. The family ate fresh fruits and vegetables and rarely ate bread, pasta, or processed foods. When she left home for her first year at college, the only food available was cafeteria-style institutional food, heavily processed, nutrient-deficient, and white-flour-based. In Melanie's words, her diet consisted of "bread, waffles, and starch."

As a young child, Melanie's immune system never developed tolerance to gluten-containing foods. When her lifelong diet changed drastically during her freshman college year, her immune system responded to the presence of the new foreign protein—gluten. Her digestive system overloaded with gluten-containing grains and her immune system mounted a rapid and devastating defense against these foreign proteins.

Every one of her major health problems began after she encountered a gluten-centric diet. "If years ago I had been diagnosed with celiac disease instead of an intestinal infection, I would never have developed all those drug allergies, and many other problems could have been avoided." This is the great difficulty with gluten intolerance and celiac disease. These disorders can masquerade as autoimmune, rheumatologic, and metabolic diseases.

Melanie's medical history and experiences are both unusual and familiar. Unusual in terms of the variety and extent of her medical problems, and familiar to the many Americans and Europeans who live with gluten intolerance and celiac disease. The best news, is that there is a cure.

Living in a Wheat-Centric World

Wheat is everywhere. It's in your bread, your biscuits, your breakfast, and in your beer. We live in a wheat-centric world.

Wheat has provided great benefits for humankind. Entire civilizations have been built around this abundant and important crop. Primitive relatives of modern wheat have been found in excavations estimated to be 10,000 years old. Wheat was grown in Egypt, India, and China 5,000 years ago, is hardy, and adapts well to harsh conditions, which enabled humans to expand their range and thrive in otherwise inhospitable regions. The wind-swept plains of Middle America's Oklahoma, Kansas, and Nebraska are natural planting grounds for wheat, as are regions as far-flung as the Mongolian steppes.

Wheat is a staple of the global economy. The United States Department of Agriculture's Foreign Agricultural Services states that 715 million metric tons of it was harvested worldwide in 2014. Wheat futures are an important commodity on the Chicago Board of Trade and a staple of the kitchen table. Americans consume more wheat than any other single food, and it accounts for 20% of the calories of the world's population, but there is a dark side to wheat.

For the many millions who are gluten intolerant, consumption of wheat can lead to serious health problems. Tens of millions, possibly 40-50 million Americans are gluten intolerant, and most do not realize it. Similar numbers of Europeans are also gluten intolerant.

What does it mean to be gluten intolerant? Remarkably, despite the long history of wheat in our global society, the human body cannot digest its primary proteins known in combination as gluten, which are what make wheat, wheat. Humans lack the necessary enzymes to break down gluten proteins into amino acids, the building blocks of protein and we don't have the genetic information necessary to build gluten-digesting enzymes. These undigested gluten proteins pass through the gastrointestinal system of some people without causing any harm, but for those who are gluten intolerant, gluten proteins can mean major health problems.

Gluten in History

Wheat cultivation began in approximately 10,000 years ago, in a region incorporating present day Israel, Iraq, western Iran, southeastern Turkey, and Syria, known as the Fertile Crescent. Wheat reached Great Britain, Ireland, and Spain approximately 5,000 years ago. Originally wheat species were genetically diverse, but grains that were genetically uniform produced more stable crops and higher yields. In addition, people selected the grains that worked best for bread making because they possessed a glue-like property that helped dough stick together. The structural proteins that produce yields of sticky dough are known as gluten.

As a result, gluten-containing wheat became the standard wheat crop. Today, all wheat consumed around the world contains gluten. The protein in barley and rye is also predominantly gluten. If wheat is such a prevalent part of our diets, why are so many people gluten intolerant? Why aren't tens of millions of people intolerant to chicken or apples or spinach? These foods are all important parts of many families' regular meals. If exposure is the problem, why is gluten such a common culprit and why does it cause so many disorders? The answers to these important questions, although theoretical, are deeply complex.

Gluten Intolerance and a Competitive Advantage

In the United States today, life expectancy for men is approximately 76 years and for women, approximately 81 years. Only 100 years ago life expectancy in the U.S. was approximately 47 years for both sexes. In the middle ages in Europe, 30 years of age represented a good long life. The dramatic gains in life expectancy are the result of advances in the practice of medicine, specifically the development of antibiotics and vaccines, as well as widespread clean water and sanitation.

Prior to the era of modern medicine, infections were the main causes of death. One part of a useful working theory for why gluten intolerance is on the rise suggests that in previous eras the vast majority of people died before they had time to manifest symptoms of intolerance. Many infants and children perished owing to a broad array of infectious diseases: influenza, pneumonia, whooping cough, diphtheria, measles, mumps, smallpox, and polio. Infants and children were also highly susceptible to death from gastrointestinal infections from contaminated water supplies and lack of sanitation.

In the case of ever-present gastrointestinal infections, those who survived attacks of colitis, jejunitis, gastroenteritis, cholera, dysentery, and chronic diarrhea were able to confer this important competitive advantage to their offspring, passing the genes responsible for this mysterious cloak of protection along to the next generation.

The children of those who survived were better able to recover from deadly gastrointestinal infections, and transmitted these survival characteristics to their children. What was the likely source of this competitive advantage that was now being selected by the formidable machinery of evolution? The probable source is the mechanism of gluten intolerance itself.

As we've discussed, humans never developed the capacity to digest gluten. Wheat was not a food source when Homo sapiens became a distinct species in eastern Africa approximately 200,000 years ago. Wheat arrived relatively late on the scene, about 10,000 years ago. Our enzymatic system, based on our genetic code, has never caught up. What happens when we digest gluten-containing bread or wheat products? We can only partially digest gluten, breaking it down into large fragments.

In many people, these fragments provoke an immune reaction culminating in an inflammatory response. The focus of the inflammation is the lining of the gastrointestinal tract, specifically the lining of the small intestine. Many serious problems can develop if such an intestinal inflammation becomes widespread, but in most people the inflammatory changes are low-grade and do not cause symptoms, but in every person the intestinal inflammation has a side benefit. The inflammation provoked by gluten fragments confers a relative resistance to gastrointestinal infections which provided a competitive advantage. Those who developed inflammation were better able to survive, so the genes for gluten intolerance persisted and spread in the population. As a result, large numbers of people in the modern world are gluten intolerant. Serious problems are likely to develop in persons in whom gluten intolerance provokes more than a low-grade immune response.

Gluten Intolerance Is a Cause of Many Diseases and Disorders

As we shall see, people with clinically significant gluten intolerance experience a wide variety of symptoms and diseases. As the inflammation of the small intestine worsens, the person is less able to absorb nutrients, including proteins, vitamins, and minerals. This is known as malabsorption syndrome, and the long-term result is a lengthy list of digestive disorders and metabolic diseases stemming from a lack of proper nutrition.

Gluten-intolerance is also associated with a variety of autoimmune disorders, which may be linked to the immune reaction provoked by gluten. A person with an autoimmune disease makes antibodies that destroy their own tissues. These antibodies directed against the "self" are called autoantibodies. If they target joints, the person develops rheumatoid arthritis. If they target the kidneys, the nervous system, the skin, and/or the heart, the diagnosis may be systemic lupus erythematosus (SLE), simply referred to as lupus. If they target the muscles, the person develops polymyositis or dermatomyositis. If they target the thyroid, the person develops Hashimoto's thyroiditis. Gluten-intolerance may also play a role in autism, attention deficit hyperactivity disorder (ADHD), and schizophrenia, although these links are not yet fully understood.

The bottom line is that the symptoms of gluten-intolerance are highly variable. Diseases that may be linked to gluten intolerance include:

- Attention deficit disorder
- Autism
- Diabetes
- Fibromyalgia
- Hashimoto's thyroiditis (an autoimmune endocrinopathy)
- Iron deficiency anemia
- Lupus (systemic lupus erythematosus)
- Mixed connective tissue disorder
- Neurologic disorders
- Osteoarthritis
- Osteopenia (loss of bone mass)
- Osteoporosis
- Pseudogout
- Rheumatoid arthritis
- Schizophrenia
- Sjögren's syndrome (a multisystem autoimmune disorder)

Gluten intolerance may be responsible for many unexplained symptoms including:

- Bloating and abdominal pain
- Chronic fatigue
- Diarrhea or constipation
- Failure to thrive
- Frequent colds and infections
- Frequent headaches
- Infertility
- Mood disorders including apathy and lethargy
- Recurrent fetal loss
- Short stature
- Vitamin deficiencies
- Weakness and fatigue

In many cases, persons with gluten intolerance do not have gastrointestinal-related symptoms. Instead, they have symptoms of the related diseases, such as attention deficit disorder or rheumatoid arthritis. It can be difficult for a physician to correctly identify the underlying cause of a person's ongoing symptoms and at present most affected individuals go undiagnosed.

Most physicians are not trained to recognize the signs and symptoms of gluten intolerance. If a person is experiencing chronic joint pain, a physician would have to be very well informed to include gluten intolerance in her list of diagnostic possibilities. Likewise, if a child demonstrates early signs of autism, the large majority of pediatricians and pediatric psychologists would not consider gluten intolerance as a possible primary cause.

This lack of awareness among physicians and the public too often leads to misdiagnosis, inappropriate and ineffective treatment, significant decreases in quality of life, and persistent and aggravated symptoms. For example, if a person complains of fatigue, weakness, muscle aches, and joint pain, their family physician might order blood tests for rheumatoid arthritis and lupus. If these tests are negative the patient could be referred to a rheumatologist. If the rheumatologist is not familiar with gluten intolerance and celiac disease, he might offer a diagnosis of mixed connective tissue disorder and prescribe a course of steroid medication. If the real cause isn't corrected, symptoms will continue and may worsen, and the side effects of inappropriate medication may create additional problems.

Quality of life is a day-to-day concern for those affected by gluten intolerance. Some people suffer from debilitating diarrhea while others have bloating and abdominal pain. The fatigue, weakness, muscle aches, and joint pains associated with gluten intolerance may be profound. Such persons may dread getting up in the morning because they know the day will bring prolonged periods of discomfort, pain, and stress.

Quality of life can deteriorate further following an ineffective interaction with a physician. If the physician does not have gluten intolerance or celiac disease in mind, they may choose to go down a diagnostic pathway that appears to fit the patient's symptoms, but misses the underlying cause. Much time is then wasted in specialist referrals, unnecessary diagnostic tests, and prescription of ineffective and potentially harmful medications. Patients naturally get their hopes up when they begin receiving some kind of treatment, but the ultimate persistence of very uncomfortable symptoms can be devastating.

Heightened awareness of gluten intolerance and celiac disease is the key to effective diagnosis. Family physicians as well as specialists in all fields see what they look for and recognize what they know. Habits of thought are useful, but they restrict the ability to create new associations and identify situations that don't fit into previously established patterns. Correctly identifying gluten intolerance and/or celiac disease as the cause of rheumatic, immunologic, and endocrine diseases will have wide-ranging benefits for millions of people. To achieve this goal, The National Institutes of Health Consensus Statement on Celiac Disease calls for education of physicians, nurses, dietitians, and the public. This book is intended to meet that goal and raise awareness and understanding of gluten intolerance and celiac disease with the public and those entrusted with the health of patients seeking treatment.

When to Suspect Gluten Intolerance and Celiac Disease

Gluten intolerance and celiac disease may show classical symptoms, but these disorders are also great mimickers. Physicians need to have a clear working knowledge of gluten intolerance and celiac disease. Also critical is an understanding of the association and relationship of gluten intolerance and celiac disease with many important disease categories including autoimmune disorders, endocrine diseases, neuropsychiatric conditions, infertility, and malignancy.

Diagnosing gluten intolerance and celiac disease in infants and young children is relatively straightforward. Affected children in these age groups generally have diarrhea and abdominal bloating. Their physical development will lag behind expected standards regarding height and weight. Such delayed development is known as failure to thrive. Vomiting, constipation, and irritability may also be observed. In infants and young children, such an array of signs and symptoms should place gluten intolerance and celiac disease at the top of the list of suspected causes.

In adults the diagnosis is much less clear. Adults with gluten intolerance and celiac disease classically have diarrhea, abdominal bloating, and abdominal pain, but in the last 10 years diarrhea has been the main complaint in less than 50% of patients. The real difficulty in diagnosis occurs when abdominal symptoms are entirely absent. In such circumstances, a high index of suspicion is needed. In adults, gluten intolerance and celiac disease may also be suspected in cases of autoimmune disease, endocrine disorders, iron deficiency anemia, neurologic disorders, osteoporosis, and/or problems with fertility. The list of diseases associated with any of these disorders is extensive, however gluten intolerance and celiac disease should always be considered, even when other causes have been identified. Many people with celiac disease are seeking treatment for a wide variety of common symptoms, none of which is particularly suggestive of celiac disease. It is important for physicians to question their assumptions, continue to question the evidence, and seek answers beyond those that are obvious. Persistence of symptoms even with treatment is the single most important clue that the diagnosis is incomplete, inaccurate, or both.

Despite its unfamiliarity to many physicians, celiac disease is a common disorder, affecting approximately one in every 100 adults. In the majority of these individuals, gluten intolerance and celiac disease remain undiagnosed, emphasizing the need for knowledge and awareness.

Accurate information empowers people to take positive action on their own behalf. The modern improving medical environment focuses on a doctor–patient partnership. Doctors do not "know everything" and patients can bring a lot to the relationship, provided they are well informed. With respect to gluten intolerance and celiac disease, knowledge and awareness are the key elements in identifying a correct diagnosis.

It is important for patients to seek help from a doctor who is well versed on celiac disease and the correlation to other autoimmune diseases. An important question for any patient to ask a doctor is "What conditions are on your differential list?" In today's harried medical environment, time is at a premium, but time constraints cannot be used as justification for failing to thoroughly analyze a patient's particular circumstances. Physicians need to be reminded to stop and think. Asking, "What conditions are on your differential list" will do just that.

Skilled physicians are trained to arrive at a diagnostic conclusion by considering all the evidence. The process involves eliminating suspected disorders that might be responsible for a given set of symptoms. The doctor develops a short list of conditions, usually five or six, and rank-orders them. The top three diseases on the list will probably account for more than 95% of cases and the remaining two or three are uncommon conditions that must be considered until they're eliminated.

For example, unexplained persistent fever, joint pain and joint swelling, weakness, and fatigue could be caused by rheumatoid arthritis, lupus, reactive arthritis, infectious disease, and malignancy. The complete list is much longer, and more than one of these conditions can be present, complicating the analysis. The important point is to consider a group of suspected conditions rather than jumping to an easy conclusion and focusing on the top one or two. Experienced clinicians can do all this in their heads. They've gone through these parameters hundreds of times, but it's easy to forget to be rigorous. Asking "What conditions are on your differential list" reminds your doctor to slow down and consider unlikely alternatives. You can even be more direct and say, "Please be sure to consider gluten intolerance and celiac disease in your list of differential diagnoses."

Homo glutenicus

The birth of *Homo glutenicus*, or gluten cautious individuals has been in the making for over 10 years. *Homo glutenicus* is the mass of people creating a community that is influencing the food industry for more gluten free options, the medical community for more education and awareness, and society for more acceptance and support for individuals who are embarking on a gluten free lifestyle

The good news is that awareness of gluten intolerance and its close association with a wide variety of serious conditions is developing critical mass. There are dozens of well written web sites focusing on gluten intolerance and many more offering lifestyle tips and gluten free recipes. A number of good books on gluten intolerance have been published recently, and articles on gluten intolerance and a gluten-free lifestyle appear regularly in blogs, newspapers, and healthy living magazines. The gluten free revolution is happening now.

In this book, we will explore the hidden roles that gluten and gluten intolerance play in millions of lives and discuss the science behind gluten intolerance and the evidence showing how gluten intolerance may be linked to a variety of major health problems, from arthritis to autism. Most importantly, we will present and describe a surprisingly simple, safe, and inexpensive cure: a gluten free diet. Along the way, we will share stories of real people who, like Melanie, have transformed their lives by eliminating gluten.

Gluten and Autoimmune Diseases

The Path to a Cure

Susan Perry loved playing sports. She joined a softball league when she was eight and added soccer when she was ten. In 1989 when she turned 13, Susan started running cross-country track for her middle school's team, and continued with all three sports throughout high school. At her Division II college, athletics were a lot more competitive than in high school, so Susan decided to give up team sports for a year or two. When her track friends recommended mountain biking, Susan discovered a new way to have fun.

Always an organizer, Susan launched an informal cycling club with friends who got together a few times each month at different trailheads, setting out in the early morning and regrouping at a local brunch hangout after a raucous 20K or 30K ride. Susan learned how to support her mountain-biker lifestyle by doing strength training for her upper body and soon discovered that she was in the best shape of her life.

Susan concluded that strength training had made the difference. She did some research and found out about cross-training, learning that different kinds of exercise made her a better cyclist, and mountain-biking made her stronger. Susan told everyone she knew about her discovery, sometimes finding that she was preaching to the converted, but often her information was new to people who caught her enthusiasm and became excited themselves.

Susan had found a niche in an area where she had great interest and provided a lot of value for people. She switched her major from psychology to physical education and started giving talks on sports and fitness at local high schools and community centers. At first, she was nervous about public speaking, but she was highly motivated and an expert in her subject and soon blossomed into a confident, entertaining, and informative presenter.

Susan gave a few talks each month, except those months when she had finals. When senior year approached Susan considered graduate school, thinking she'd get a M.S. in exercise science. She was working hard, having some fun, and meeting interesting people. One evening after a high school talk, a woman gave her a business card. Susan glanced at the glossy rectangle. The woman was a producer for a local TV news station. They met for coffee the next morning and the producer invited Susan to do a few spots for the station's early evening news show. "I'm not making any promises," the producer cautioned. "Let's see how it goes." The next day Susan's three-mile bike ride to class never felt easier.

The tapings were scheduled to begin in four weeks. Susan shared her excitement with her classmates, neighbors, and family. Everyone was happy for her until a few days after her meeting with the producer, when a strange thing happened while sitting in an afternoon anatomy lecture.

Susan noticed that her entire body began to feel sore. A few hours later she got a fever, and the next morning her legs felt so weak she could barely get out of bed. The fever came and went during the next seven days. Susan would feel fine for a few hours, then grew flushed and sweaty. The muscle weakness in her legs spread to her back and neck. By the end of the week, she felt very fatigued and weak all over. Her sleep wasn't restful and overnight fevers made her bed sheets damp. Susan became concerned and a little frightened, so when her parents insisted she see a doctor, Susan agreed, little realizing her life was about to change—and not for the better.

The enzyme **creatine phosphokinase (CPK)** is found in skeletal muscle, the heart, and the brain. CPK participates in the storage and use of energy in metabolic processes. Elevated CPK levels suggest muscle damage or injury, a heart attack, or a brain injury such as a stroke.

In addition, elevated CPK is an early finding in both polymyositis and dermatomyositis.

In 1996, at age 20, Susan Perry was diagnosed with polymyositis and dermatomyositis—two closely related autoimmune diseases that affect the muscles and the skin. She was experiencing profound muscle weakness, chills, and fatigue. These disturbing symptoms would improve and worsen, back and forth, for no reason Susan could understand. When her symptoms became significantly worse, Susan saw a rheumatologist and was hospitalized with high fever and high levels of creatine phosphokinase (CPK) in her blood. Elevated CPK means that muscle cells and muscle tissue are being damaged or destroyed. Injury or cell death causes leakage of the cell's enzymes into the surrounding fluid. These biochemicals are then absorbed into the bloodstream. For Susan, the elevated CPK values meant that extensive damage was being done to her muscles.

Her rheumatologist prescribed high doses of intravenous methylprednisolone as the first attempt to treat her autoimmune disease. Methylprednisolone, a particularly effective immunosuppressive medication, is a corticosteroid often used to combat out-of-control immune system reactions. Susan was hospitalized for a week. Her fever lessened as a result of treatment, but her muscle weakness persisted.

For the next three years Susan continued to take oral prednisone as well as methotrexate, a drug used primarily in cancer treatment, but also in the treatment of autoimmune diseases. In 1999, aggravated symptoms returned, and Susan was again hospitalized for high fever and severe muscle weakness. Her CPK level was 14,000; almost 70 times higher than maximum normal values. A muscle biopsy confirmed inflammation characteristic of polymyositis and dermatomyositis. Dosages of both prednisone and methotrexate were increased and Susan's fever, chills, and muscle weakness improved, but she "never really regained complete strength."

In 2001, Susan's CPK levels rose steadily to 10,000 and in May 2001, she was hospitalized for severe abdominal pain. The diagnosis was gastroenteritis and "early hepatitis." Gastrointestinal ulcers were discovered and attributed to her long-term use of high doses of prednisone, so her dose of prednisone was lowered and CellCept was prescribed as an additional immunosuppressive drug. CellCept is mainly used in kidney transplantation cases to reduce the likelihood of transplant rejection.

Susan continued to develop new disorders. In 2002, a bone density exam showed mild osteopenia, a loss of bone density caused by, in this case, chronic prednisone use. She also had "lots of breathing problems," a probable side-effect of CellCept. In 2003, Susan had a biking accident and felt she was "getting weaker." Her CPK level was 3000. She had discontinued prednisone because of its side effects, but she still took CellCept. Her rheumatologist also prescribed Enbrel, another drug used in the treatment of autoimmune diseases like rheumatoid arthritis and ankylosing spondylitis. Enbrel was not particularly effective. Susan's CPK level continued to climb to 6000, so she decided not to go back to prednisone.

Prednisone is a synthetic corticosteroid medication derived from cortisone. Prednisone is an inactive drug. It is activated by the liver in a process that produces prednisolone. In other words, prednisolone is the biologically active form of prednisone. In certain individuals, administration of the biologically active form has a more beneficial effect.

In mid-2003 when she was 27 years old, Susan decided to stop all medications because of their side effects. Within two months she was so physically weak that she fell forward and hit her head on the bathroom tiles, resulting in a concussion. Her muscle weakness was so profound she started using a walker and her CPK level was 12,000, so she resumed Enbrel, but it had no effect. Her CPK levels reached an alarming 17,500 in September 2003.

Her doctors were puzzled about what to do next. Prednisolone, the active metabolite of prednisone, seemed a good idea. CPK levels decreased to 7500 on it.

In early 2004, Neoral was added to Susan's medication regime.

Neoral (cyclosporine) is an immunosuppressive drug used in psoriasis and autoimmune diseases like rheumatoid arthritis. Neoral was more effective than Enbrel and Susan felt "more balanced." As a result, she was able to discontinue using her walker, but was soon admitted to the hospital with severe abdominal pain.

At this point, overwhelmed by so many effects, Susan was "pretty much against all medications—even if it meant death." She didn't care and ceased all medications in July 2004 and searched for alternatives. She learned about vegan diets and began a "complete vegan diet" in September of that year. She immediately lost a lot of weight which was not a good thing because she had trouble maintaining her weight, but in December, Susan's CPK level was 2500, lower than it had been in more than a year. "My vegan diet was impacting my CPK," she said." Additionally, a new muscle biopsy showed reduced inflammation, another very good sign.

Susan remained on the vegan diet and by March 2005, her CPK level had dropped to 1600, a remarkable result. Her rheumatologist said this was "coincidental" and not related to her dietary modifications and strongly recommended that Susan undergo plasmapheresis, an invasive procedure with many potential side effects. In plasmapheresis, the patient's blood is removed a batch at a time, using a needle or a catheter. The antibody-containing plasma is separated from the red and white blood cells, and the plasma-free cells are returned to the patient to remove disease-causing autoantibodies, offering short-term improvement in their symptoms and a chance to better respond to immunosuppressive medication. Plasmapheresis can lead to significant complications.

Susan's rheumatologist said she "would be cured," but Susan honestly believed she was healing herself with her diet. Owing to her doctor's strong recommendation and family pressure, Susan agreed to undergo the procedure in March 2005 which Susan remembered, saying, "Plasmapheresis was one of the most horrifying experiences of my life." A semi-permanent catheter was inserted and Susan received treatment three times per week for six weeks.

She weighed 116 pounds at the start of plasmapheresis and weighed 99 pounds at the end of the six-week treatment, but her CPK levels, which had been 1400, were down to 120. Susan was uncertain as to whether the improvement was because of diet, the treatment, or both. Despite a good outcome, Susan experienced ongoing diarrhea, vomiting, and loss of appetite. An additional three months of plasmapheresis was recommended, but Susan opposed it. Her rheumatologist predicted an immediate elevation of CPK and said Susan would be sicker than ever.

Susan refused further interventions, but continued her strict diet. By November, her CPK had risen to 950, went back down to 180 by January 2006. Her CPK level settled at 80 U/L and has remained there permanently.

In July 2006, Susan experienced more abdominal pain which no one could figure out. A gastroenterologist proposed a motility issue caused by polymyositis and an endoscopy showed upper gastrointestinal ulcers, but these came from Susan's history of prednisone. She never received a conclusive diagnosis on her abdominal symptoms, but she continued to get stronger. Her chronic muscle weakness and inflammation seemed to have resolved and she was able to exercise for the first time in many years, feeling "invincible" until January 2007 when she was hospitalized again for severe abdominal pain.

An internist diagnosed a protein deficiency and recommended salmon as a good protein source. Susan took this advice, went off her vegan diet, and gained some weight, but her abdominal pain persisted. During the summer of 2007 her boyfriend Rick developed knee, shoulder, and wrist pain that was diagnosed as arthritis. He consulted with our clinic, and underwent extensive laboratory testing that revealed a high probability of gluten intolerance. Rick was advised to try a gluten-free diet and his joint pains quickly resolved. He felt so much better in such a short period of time, he termed the improvement "miraculous."

As a result of Rick's recovery, Susan made an appointment with our clinic when her abdominal pain became intolerable and she was experiencing chronic diarrhea, once again losing a lot of weight. After laboratory testing Susan was diagnosed with gluten intolerance and placed on a strict gluten-free diet and in December 2007 her abdominal pain went away immediately.

Fast forward to June 2009. "All my muscle weakness and fatigue are gone," Susan said. Her CPK levels remained normal and all her other blood work was normal. Susan has weighed 116 pounds since she started the gluten-free diet and does one hour of exercise three times per week. "I feel strong," she added, laughing. "This is what happens when you give up Dunkin' Donuts."

Regarding the gluten-free diet, Susan said, "You have to make a decision that will change your life forever. Once you see the results the decision is easy. Originally you think you won't be able to survive, but you have a choice of living in misery and pain, or the option of food without gluten and having a beautiful life. Many of us go through years of suffering, wanting to die, but the suffering can end and a cure is available."

Autoimmune Diseases: What Do They Mean for Me?

Receiving a diagnosis of an autoimmune disease is akin to receiving a life sentence. You're never cured and you have to make the best of it. There are treatments, but no medical cures. A person is on medications for life. The two main goals of drug therapy are to reduce pain and inflammation and suppress the over reactive immune system. Prolonged drug therapy can lead to side effects, some of which can be life-threatening.

A person with an autoimmune disease is in a tough situation. Medications are needed to control the symptoms and the disease itself, but the medications frequently create new problems. Similar tradeoffs play a role in the treatment of other chronic diseases like cancer and heart disease. The key question is: are there additional approaches and actions to supplement traditional medical strategies?

The answer is yes, and we're going to discuss these critical solutions, but first we will explore autoimmune diseases and their impact on patients, so we can put these solutions into context and understand how they work.

What Is Autoimmunity and How Does It Cause So Many Problems?

Autoimmunity means that your immune system mistakes your own tissues and cells for foreign ones. The function of the immune system is to attack and destroy substances that are not-self, which means that autoimmune diseases target your own living architecture. Specific autoimmune diseases attack specific organs and tissues. Here is a list of the most common autoimmune disorders and their target organs and tissues:

- Hashimoto's thyroiditis attacks the thyroid
- Lupus affects the kidneys, heart, joints, blood vessels, and skin
- Multiple sclerosis affects the nervous system
- Polymyositis attacks muscles
- Rheumatoid arthritis attacks joints and associated soft tissues
- Scleroderma affects the skin, heart, kidneys, and lungs
- Sjögren's syndrome affects glands that produce tears and saliva

There are many other forms of autoimmune disease. Their common factor is the presence of autoantibodies, that is, antibodies directed against the self. The causes of these disorders are unknown, but various mechanisms have been considered. For example, many persons have a genetic predisposition to develop autoantibodies. Additionally, several environmental factors have been proposed, including exposure to toxic metals and toxic chemicals. Infectious agents, including bacteria and viruses, have also been implicated. Significant stress and trauma have also been identified in many cases. We can reasonably conclude that autoimmune diseases are caused by a combination of factors.

Autoimmune diseases are difficult and traditional medical treatment is challenging. The immune system, even a faulty one, is necessary for life. You can't shut it off for obvious reasons. Half-measures are usually taken. Doctors prescribe immunosuppressive medications such as steroids, which suppress some immune activity, but leave enough immune function to allow the patient to survive. This is a fine line and most patients live with compromised immune systems making them susceptible to infection. They are often weak and fatigued, owing to an ineffective immune response.

The same problem exists in the treatment of cancer patients. Standard therapy for aggressive cancers includes surgery, chemotherapy, and/or radiation. Over the years, radiation has become more precisely targeted, but chemotherapy remains an all-or-nothing approach. These drugs kill rapidly reproducing cells, which makes sense because aggressive cancer cells reproduce quickly. Their growth is unchecked by normal regulatory mechanisms so they have to be killed, but the drugs kill all rapidly dividing cells, including "good" ones which is why cancer patients on chemotherapy lose their hair, their appetite, and have nausea, vomiting, and diarrhea. Cells lining the digestive tract, as well as hair follicles, are all rapidly reproducing cells. Chemotherapy patients may become anemic and their immune systems are depressed because both red and white blood cells are produced by cell lines that reproduce rapidly.

Like treatment for autoimmune diseases, cancer therapy also draws a fine line between the goods and harms associated with treatment. The patient is given enough drugs to help slow cancer growth, but not so much that it will kill them.

Treatment for these chronic diseases is not the same as treatment for acute disorders like infections. With an infection, the initial problem is to identify the cause. The second problem is to discover a drug that will kill the bacteria, virus, or parasite. Historically in an infection there is almost always a one-to-one relationship between the microorganism causing the problem and an effective medication such as an antibiotic. Also, for the majority of infections there is usually a direct relationship between treatment and cure. Historically, provision of medication results in a cure, but for cancer and autoimmune diseases, neither of these direct one-to-one relationships exists.

Treatment of autoimmune diseases is especially difficult as the immune mechanisms that have gone awry cannot be directly accessed. The immune system is complex and its functioning involves every other system, so even if new research identifies access points that can be manipulated with drugs (which will be at least 20 years away), the side effects are likely to be substantial. At present, the best that can be done is to suppress the immune system which is a temporary fix associated with serious side effects.

Traditional medical methods involving treatment with drugs have limited benefits. A holistic approach targeted at the underlying mechanisms of autoimmune diseases appears to have more probability of success. Holistic medicine is described as integrative medicine that addresses the individual as a whole organism. It involves lifestyle modifications, including eliminating environmental triggers that provoke autoimmune responses. Eliminating environmental triggers enables the patient's immune system to reset to normal and symptoms begin to resolve. Additional aspects of a holistic approach include medical treatment and medication as necessary, regular exercise, an overall healthful diet, and sufficient rest. By providing a more optimal external and internal environment, integrative or holistic medicine assists the body to heal itself.

The first step in designing an effective holistic treatment for autoimmune diseases is to identify a likely environmental trigger. Current research points to gluten proteins as a common causative factor.

Gluten Intolerance and Autoimmune Diseases

We have learned that food can influence both immune and inflammatory responses, and it can lead to the development of rheumatic and autoimmune diseases. Gluten proteins are one of the most common causes of such responses. In genetically susceptible individuals, gluten proteins are capable of triggering a broad spectrum of inflammatory and immune responses. As we've seen, 40% of Americans and Western Europeans are genetically susceptible to gluten intolerance and gluten-associated diseases.

In those who are susceptible, large gluten protein fragments provoke an immune reaction within the small intestine causing a cascade of inflammatory reactions. The biochemicals produced by these reactions circulate throughout the body, and can initiate immune responses in many different regions. Some of these immune responses may be directed against the body's own tissues, establishing the presence of an autoimmune disease.

Celiac disease often goes undetected for years. Research shows that the signs and symptoms of autoimmune disorders may be the first clues identifying the presence of underlying celiac disease. The duration of exposure to gluten may be a key factor in the development of autoimmune diseases associated with celiac disease.

Gluten Intolerance and Autoimmune Diseases — The Genetic and Autoantibody Connection

Immunologic studies of patients with celiac disease show many features associated with autoimmune disease. Features common to both diseases include:

- Characteristic white blood cell proliferation
- Invasion of white blood cells in affected organs

- Presence of specific autoantibodies (anti-single-stranded DNA and anti-double-stranded DNA)
- Provocation of inflammatory mechanisms by specific immunologic agents

Patients with celiac disease and those with autoimmune disorders have numerous immunologic agents in common, further suggesting a link between the two conditions. These agents are known as human leukocyte antigens (HLAs).

One such antigen, HLA DQ2, plays an important role in gluten intolerance/celiac disease. Each HLA subtype is capable of recognizing and binding to a specific foreign protein. The HLA and foreign protein binding-pair form what is known as a "complex." The creation of this complex signals a specific type of white blood cell, a T cell that initiates an immune response. In people with celiac disease, HLA DQ2 specifically binds to gluten, and the resulting complex triggers T cells located in the small intestine, leading to inflammation. Gluten intolerance represents the entire sequence of events that results from this HLA DQ2 – gluten – T cell inflammatory interaction.

HLA DQ2 is found in 95% of patients with celiac disease and in many patients with lupus, again suggesting a link between gluten intolerance and autoimmune diseases. The ability to produce HLA DQ2 is a hereditary trait.

The amount of time a genetically predisposed individual is exposed to gluten has been shown to be directly correlated with the risk of developing an autoimmune disease. A large multicenter trial conducted in Italy studied more than 900 patients with celiac disease. The prevalence of autoimmune disorders in this group was 14%, compared to a prevalence of 2.8% in 1268 controls. Additionally, the prevalence of autoimmune diseases increased in patients with celiac disease the longer it remained undiagnosed, in other words, the longer these patients were exposed to gluten.

In patients in whom celiac disease was diagnosed before the age of two, only 5% had an associated autoimmune disorder. In marked contrast, in patients who were older than age 20 before receiving a diagnosis of celiac disease, 34% had an associated autoimmune disease. Of the study patients with celiac disease, 36 (4%) also had type 1 diabetes, 32 (3.5%) had dermatitis herpetiformis, 12 (1.3%)

had mixed connective tissue disease, 12 (1.3%) had autoimmune thyroiditis, 10 (1.1%) had autoimmune hepatitis, and 4 (0.4%) had cerebellar ataxia.

In **cerebellar ataxia** the person has a significant impairment or lack of muscular coordination. The cerebellum is the part of the brain responsible for coordinating muscular movement. Cerebellar ataxia is a form of neurologic dysfunction.

Overall, the prevalence of autoimmune disease in young adult and adolescent patients with celiac disease is much higher than the general population.

Of considerable significance is that symptoms of autoimmune diseases can be improved with a gluten-free diet. This effect has been documented in cases of juvenile rheumatoid arthritis and cerebellar ataxia, proving that in genetically predisposed individuals, gluten is a potential trigger for a wide range of autoimmune disorders.

A Look Under the Hood: The Development of Celiac Disease

A number of critical questions have puzzled researchers in the fields of gastroenterology (the study of diseases of the digestive system), immunology, and rheumatology (the study of diseases of the musculoskeletal system) for many years.

- Why might there be any relationship at all between gluten intolerance and autoimmune disorders?
- What is the nature of the immunologic reaction to gluten?
- Why do people develop such profound symptoms and become sick as a result of eating foods containing wheat, barley, or rye?
- Why do only some people who are genetically susceptible to gluten intolerance develop symptoms?

These questions have been investigated for decades, primarily in Europe, and many fascinating and highly complex answers have been provided. Immunology itself is a complicated field with multiple interactions among components and participating factors. In attempting to answer these questions, immunologists have frequently lost their way during the last 50 years, but persistence has paid off and numerous breakthroughs have been achieved in the last two decades.

As gluten is not digestible by humans, our enzymes can only break it into large fragments which may be acted upon by a particular common enzyme found in many locations throughout the body, including the cells residing below the inner lining of the small intestine. After years of research, this enzyme was identified as tissue transglutaminase (tTG).

tTG is localized to a layer of cells in the small intestine known as the *lamina propria,* an inner lining layer and the major site of immunologic damage in celiac disease. Excellent scientific work has been done tracking down the enzyme tTG. These findings interlock and confirm each other.

tTG has many functions in the body, including assisting in wound healing and the creation of the intercellular matrix, the gel-like substance that holds cells together. In the small intestine, tTG may interact with gluten protein fragments, causing a biochemical change (deamidation) that primes gluten fragments to set off a widespread immune response.

Left on their own, these fragments wouldn't cause any problems. They'd be excreted along with the other unusable parts of the food we eat, but in genetically susceptible individuals, in combination with certain environmental factors, the interaction of gluten fragments with tTG launches an immunological chain reaction.

Why do only a small proportion of people who are genetically susceptible to gluten intolerance develop symptoms? Approximately 40% of individuals have the gene that leads to the construction of HLA DQ2, antigen-displaying proteins present in the majority of those genetically susceptible to gluten intolerance and celiac disease. In addition, all the other biochemical factors in the gluten intolerance immune response, the tTG enzyme, HLA helper T cells, and B cells, are all present in genetically susceptible individuals as well.

The key to understanding this difficult question is that genetics are not the only important factor. How the genetic sequence is expressed is important, but the internal environment of the individual also represents a critical dynamic.

Two persons may share an identical genetic sequence for a certain characteristic, but only one might show the specific characteristic. The expression of a genetic sequence depends on a highly complex set of molecular factors. Usually there are a number of feedback mechanisms involved, some enhancing and others inhibiting gene expression and protein manufacture. The internal environment of the cell tips the balance, favoring gene expression or no gene expression. Person A and person B may both have a genetic sequence coding for antigen-presenting DQ, but only person A will manufacture DQ and develop gluten intolerance as a consequence of person A's internal molecular environment.

Gluten Intolerance and Rheumatoid Arthritis

Rheumatoid arthritis (RA) is an autoimmune disease that causes chronic inflammation of joints, particularly the hands, wrist, feet, neck, hips, and knees. RA can also affect mucous membranes lining the heart and lungs. The chronic inflammation of RA causes great suffering. Affected joints are swollen, warm, painful, and stiff. RA can result in permanent deformity.

Treatment is difficult. Traditionally, RA was treated with gold compounds because of their anti-inflammatory effects, but gold accumulates in the body and is toxic. Recent advances in understanding the immune mechanisms involved in RA have led to the development of powerful medications. These newer drugs include various biologic agents such as: adalimumab (Humira), etanercept (Enbrel), infliximab (Remicade), and rituximab (Rituxan), among others. Older drugs such as methotrexate are still widely used, but all of these medications can have significant side effects.

Understanding the causes of RA has been difficult as the malady has both autoimmune and inflammatory characteristics. Current RA disease models propose multiple mechanisms. T cells (lymphocytes that mature in the thymus and play central roles in numerous immunologic processes) are important in RA, as they are in celiac disease. T cells have been identified as the driving force in RA pathology and symptoms. Research investigating RA has discovered antigen-presenting DR proteins whose presence helps explain the autoimmune aspects of the disease and suggest a genetic component to RA, as these molecules are encoded by specific DNA sites. This research might aid in understanding why RA is often found in families.

A relationship between celiac disease and RA was established several decades ago when researchers in the United Kingdom presented three case reports involving co-existing celiac disease and RA. The link involves immune complexes found in both diseases. Research shows strong associations between celiac disease and rheumatoid arthritis. Many immunologic features are common to both, suggesting interrelated causes and common elements relate to specific immunologic properties.

Many rheumatoid arthritis patients have antigen-presenting DQ as well as DR molecules. DQ-positive patients show a high responsiveness to specific autoantigens, suggesting a link between celiac disease and increased symptoms of RA. Laboratory studies also point to possible relationships between RA, gluten intolerance, and celiac disease. In transgenic mice, the presence of immune-active DQ molecules was associated with the likelihood of the mice developing rheumatoid arthritis.

A study in Italy evaluated 119 children with juvenile rheumatoid arthritis. Four (3.3%) of these children had antibodies suggesting the presence of celiac disease, a rate three times higher than that in the general population. Placing these children on gluten-free diets had startling results. One child had been below the 30th percentiles for both height and weight. After employing a gluten-free diet, she promptly improved in both categories, gaining 22 pounds and growing more than two inches within ten months. Another child's weight improved from the 50th to the 75th percentile within six months.

In both children, juvenile RA went into remission. Immunosuppressive therapy was discontinued in one child and continued at a low dosage in another. Eliminating gluten had a much greater impact on the course of the disease and the lives of these children than medical treatment alone.

We may conclude that for those who suffer from both celiac disease and rheumatoid arthritis, successful treatment of celiac disease by addressing the underlying gluten intolerance also has a positive effect on the painful and debilitating symptoms of rheumatoid arthritis.

Gluten Intolerance and Systemic Lupus Erythematosus

Systemic lupus erythematosus (SLE), or commonly referred to as lupus, is an autoimmune disease that involves multiple body systems. Lupus affects joints, kidneys, the nervous system, lungs, the skin, and additional organs and systems and is characterized by periods of worsening and improvement, known as exacerbations and remissions. During severe attacks, blood vessels may become inflamed (vasculitis). Women are affected ten times as often by lupus as men. The disease usually develops in young adults between the ages of 20 and 40. Its diagnosis is based on a broad set of signs and symptoms as well as specific blood tests. The range of signs and symptoms includes:

- Abdominal pain
- Anemia
- Fatigue
- Fever
- Hair loss
- Joint pains
- Mouth ulcers
- Skin rashes
- Weight loss

Laboratory tests may demonstrate specific autoantibodies that target a person's own DNA, but the presence of such autoantibodies is not proof that a person has lupus. There are a sizable proportion of false positive tests, in which the person has the antibody but not the disease.

Researchers and clinicians have discovered links between celiac disease and lupus. In a group of 246 patients with celiac disease, one study identified six patients who also had lupus. A rate of 2.4% is much higher than the rate of occurrence of lupus in the general population, which is 0.01–0.05%.

The diagnostic evaluation may suggest either celiac disease or lupus. Abdominal pain may be the first and only symptom of lupus, and the presence of celiac disease may represent an unusual early symptom of lupus. Characteristic autoantibodies found in celiac disease have also been identified in patients with lupus highlighting a likely connection between these complex diseases.

A recent review of the scientific literature identified 13 case reports in which celiac disease and lupus occurred in the same patient. In these cases, the most common celiac disease symptoms were diarrhea and weight loss. Iron deficiency anemia was present in 2 individuals. In another study, antinuclear antibodies (often found in people with lupus) were identified in 9% of persons with celiac disease.

Relationship between Gluten Intolerance and Autoimmune Diseases

In the absence of a proper diagnosis of gluten intolerance, susceptible individuals continue eating gluten-containing foods. Daily intake of the triggering protein causes an ongoing autoimmune and inflammatory response and the lining of an affected person's small intestine becomes chronically inflamed and irritated while their immune system becomes hypersensitive. Depending on specific genetic and environmental factors, the person's immune system may launch attacks against other organs and systems. The link between gluten intolerance and autoimmune diseases is associated with the immune system hyperactivation common to both conditions.

Gluten places a susceptible person's immune system on an inappropriately high alert, and the result can be attacks on normal, healthy tissue. Such attacks on "self" may lead to full-blown autoimmune diseases. As we have seen, gluten intolerance and celiac disease too often go undiagnosed. Physicians of all specialties need a high index of suspicion of these conditions when consulting with patients who present with autoimmune disorders.

Practical Points

You should become suspicious that your autoimmune disease may be linked to gluten intolerance if you experience persistent:

- Arthritis/joint swelling affecting predominantly wrists
- Canker sores
- Dry skin
- Frequent bouts of acne

- Frequent bouts of the yeast infection
- Hair loss
- Irritable bowel syndrome / diarrhea/constipation/bloating
- Lactose intolerance
- Low thyroid function (hypothyroidism)
- Mucosal dryness (eye dryness, mouth dryness, vaginal dryness)
- Premature (age-inappropriate) osteopenia or osteoporosis (low bone density)
- Skin rashes over shoulders and elbows

Laboratory findings that may potentially indicate the presence of gluten intolerance include:

- Low blood level of magnesium
- Low blood level of pancreatic enzymes (lipase in particular)
- Low blood level of vitamin B12
- Low ferritin and blood iron level
- Low vitamin D level

The following questionnaire focuses on gluten intolerance. If you score high enough, try a gluten-free diet for at least three months and see if your symptoms improve, then introduce something with gluten back into your diet and see how you react. If negatively, then you need to stay on a gluten-free diet.

Gluten Intolerance Self-Assessment

1. Have you experienced or are you experiencing abdominal pain?
2. Have you experienced or are you experiencing diarrhea?
3. Have you experienced or are you experiencing constipation?
4. Have you experienced or are you experiencing bloating?
5. Have you experienced or are you experiencing eye dryness?
6. Have you experienced or are you experiencing mouth dryness and thirst?
7. Have you experienced or are you experiencing poor dental health (cavities)?

8. Have you experienced or are you experiencing vitamin D deficiency?
9. Have you ever been diagnosed with osteopenia or osteoporosis (low bone density)?
10. Have you ever been diagnosed with thyroid disease?
11. Have you ever been diagnosed with fibromyalgia (chronic muscle pain)?
12. Have you ever been diagnosed with vitiligo (areas of skin pigment loss)?
13. Have you ever been diagnosed with keratosis pilaris (goose bumps over the shoulders)?
14. Have you ever been diagnosed with low iron level or iron-deficient anemia?

Scoring

Low Probability (less than 20%): 1-2 questions

Moderate Probability (50/50 chance): 3-4 questions

High Probability (over 75%): over 4 questions

For those at moderate risk, a three month trial of a gluten-free diet is recommended. After three months, reintroduce gluten to determine whether you react negatively.

For those at high risk, a gluten-free diet is strongly recommended. Getting tested for casein, soy protein, and egg albumin intolerance is recommended.

For those at very high risk, a gluten-free diet is strongly recommended. Getting tested for casein, soy protein, and egg albumin intolerance is recommended. You should consult with a gastroenterologist or rheumatologist to rule out celiac disease.

For more in depth results please take our online self-assessment at: glutenfreeremedies.com

Gluten Intolerance and Psychiatric Disorders: Autism, Schizophrenia, and ADHD

What They Said I Had

"I never knew who I was going to be when I woke up," said Beatrice Schiffer. "Was I going to feel powerful and strong, or was it going to be the kind of day when I'd feel like anyone or anything could crush me like a bug?" The self-assured 30-year-old looked down. "I was a very unhappy teenager most of the time, but once in a while the clouds would break and the sun would peep through, then I'd get excited, thinking everything was going to be OK. The relief would be huge. I'd have so much energy, I'd be bouncing off the walls. Finally, horribly, I'd come crashing down to earth. I'd crash hard and withdraw into a shell. I wouldn't let anyone in. Sooner or later I'd notice the sun was shining a little and the whole rollercoaster would start again."

Beatrice took a deep breath and continued. "I don't think I knew what was happening. Not really. I didn't think anything was wrong with me. I was just me. Teachers ignored me. I think they were just glad to have one less troublemaking kid to deal with. I used to sit in the corner of the classroom, out of the way. Weren't my parents concerned about my performance in school? Well, my Dad moved out when I was little. My Mom couldn't be bothered. She had too much on her mind."

Beatrice blinked away the darkness that seeped into her eyes, "But she was the one who took me to the doctor. I was 14. She thought I was too thin and she brought me to see this shrink. That's when all the medication started. He put me on these drugs and I've been taking them ever since. Trileptal. It's an anticonvulsant. They also use it for bipolar disorder. That's what they said I had. They said I was bipolar, but now I think I was just a plain-old, garden-variety unhappy kid." Bipolar disorder was not Beatrice's only problem. As a teenager, she suffered from symptoms of ADHD and at the age of 14, her gallbladder stopped working. She experienced deep, burning pain in her abdominal right upper quadrant characteristic of an inflamed gallbladder. The pain became severe after eating food with a high fat content. Ice cream was bad news and cheeseburgers caused excruciating pain, but removing a gallbladder when the patient is only 14 is a radical step, so her doctors hoped a modified diet would be a good solution.

The doctors naively counted on the willpower of a teenager, but Beatrice didn't always follow the diet. By the time she was 16 food in general was an issue. Not only did fatty foods cause distress, but so did almost everything else she ate. She experienced many digestive problems including lactose intolerance, abdominal pain, diarrhea alternating with constipation, and cramping. She also developed severe heartburn and difficulty swallowing, symptoms suggesting gastroesophageal reflux disorder (GERD). Unsure about what was going on, her gastroenterologist recommended surgery, so Beatrice's gallbladder was removed and the adults around her hoped for the best.

A few years later, when she arrived at college she was suffering chronic muscular pain in her legs, arms, and back. Her feet cramped at odd times, and she developed tightness and pain in the soles of her feet and Achilles tendons. During the first semester of her freshman year these muscular pains worsened. She woke up each morning feeling beaten up, and it would take all day to feel halfway normal, but by then she was on her way to bed, dreading how she'd feel when the alarm rang again at 7:00 a.m. She had been fit as a teenager, but stopped working out when she was a college freshman. "I was in so much pain I didn't want to move," she said.

Other symptoms and disorders plagued Beatrice throughout college. She developed acne and yeast infections became chronic. Her gynecologist discovered that Beatrice's estrogen and progesterone levels were dangerously low and prescribed hormone replacement therapy. At age 22, she began taking medications normally prescribed for women in their early 50s.

Eventually, she consulted an osteopath, who ordered a battery of tests and told her she had "31 food allergies and metal toxicity." He suggested she "try cutting out gluten," but Beatrice didn't take his advice. Instead, she tried a number of different specialists, each time hoping the new doctor would be the one to help her get better. A rheumatologist diagnosed fibromyalgia, but Beatrice sensed this wasn't the right explanation and she got worse. She felt profoundly fatigued every day and developed a mysterious pain on the left side of her abdomen, which was present every day.

Eventually her symptoms became so severe that she went to urgent care. While there, she fainted and later was told by a resident that she'd been found "limp and lifeless." Lab tests showed her blood electrolytes were severely depressed and she was placed on an intravenous line delivering saline and glucose.

Addison's disease is a kidney disorder affecting the adrenal glands, resulting in fatigue, muscle weakness, weight loss, dizziness, and mood disorders. These problems are caused by low adrenal hormone levels. In certain cases, Addison's disease may be caused by

A staff endocrinologist told her she had Addison's disease and was lucky to be alive, as her adrenal glands weren't manufacturing enough cortisol (corticosteroid hormone, produced by the adrenal cortex), so Beatrice was placed on hydrocortisone to restore her steroid levels.

Over the course of a year, the Addison's disease improved. Beatrice's cortisol levels returned to normal and she slowly regained energy, but in 2013, at the age of 28 she was in a car accident. Her right knee was injured in the crash and became swollen and painful. Normally, such swelling decreases within a couple of weeks, but in Beatrice's case the problems persisted for more than six weeks. She had difficulty walking, and a friend recommended she visited our clinic, the Institute for Specialized Medicine.

Reflex sympathetic dystrophy syndrome (RSDS) is caused by a traumatic injury, which involves local nerve damage. There may be intense regional pain, swelling, discoloration, coldness, and hypersensitivity. RSDS is typically characterized by severe burning pain, most often affecting one of the extremities (arms, legs, hands, or feet).

We diagnosed reflex sympathetic dystrophy in Beatrice's right knee, a rare disorder associated with inappropriate body response to trauma. Based on her medical history, we ordered a new series of tests and learned that she was both gluten intolerant and casein (milk protein) intolerant.

We recommended a gluten and dairy free diet right away. Beatrice had heard the gluten-free assessment and advice before, but ignored the recommendations. This time she took action and the results were immediate.

Her right knee improved, her persistent muscle pains lessened, and she felt stronger. Over time, maintaining her diet, Beatrice got better and better. Two years later, she said, "After years of being in and out of doctors' offices and hospitals, most of the issues I've ever had turned out to be related to my diet. All I did was eliminate gluten, dairy, and sugar and I feel fine." On the unusual occasions when she does eat food containing gluten or dairy, she said she, "feels horrible, my feet hurt, I have muscle pains, and I catch a cold".

Today, Beatrice has a better understanding of her health status than when she was younger. She understands what's happening when she experiences symptoms and no longer feels like a stick of furniture tossed around in a tornado. She knows she doesn't heal as fast as most people and doesn't recover from colds as quickly. Her delayed abilities to heal and recover from infections are related to her complex medical history. Her adrenal glands are chronically inflamed, a long-term result of her bout with Addison's disease. As a result she fatigues more easily than others, but she has learned to manage this aspect of her health. Her chronic right knee injury flares up periodically, but the pain subsides in a few days rather than several weeks. She's able to exercise, with limitations, and hopes to return to running in the near future. "As long as I keep away from gluten," she says. "I'll be OK."

Beatrice's psychiatric symptoms are also much improved. She acknowledges that she frequently had manic episodes when she was younger. She was "very emotional, my brain was foggy, and I was depressed. I know I had ADHD. I was all over the place, but I think I was just a troubled young kid, rather than someone who had bipolar disorder. That label has been very difficult to deal with."

Since adopting a gluten and dairy free diet, Beatrice has reduced her daily dose of Trileptal, the bipolar medication she began taking at age 14 by half and hasn't experienced any bipolar-like difficulties for more than two years. She no longer suffers from ADHD type symptoms and she's much calmer and more focused.

Beatrice is now 30 years old, studying traditional oriental medicine in a four-year program and feels like her life is finally back on track. "I'd given up hope of ever feeling good again," she said recently. "Who knew that going gluten-free would have all these side benefits? Gluten causes so many problems for so many people. Everyone needs to know more about this."

Gluten Intolerance and Neuropsychiatric Disorders

Since the mid-1970s, gluten intolerance and celiac disease have been associated with autism, schizophrenia, and ADHD. Not everyone with these neuropsychiatric conditions has gluten intolerance or celiac disease, and not everyone with gluten intolerance or celiac disease has autism, schizophrenia, or ADHD, but in predisposed individuals, the association is well recognized in scientific literature.

During the last 30-plus years, journal articles have reported links between autism and celiac disease or resolution of ADHD symptoms after initiation of a gluten-free diet. Similar findings have been reported in patients with schizophrenia. For the most part these articles consist of case studies of one or a few individuals or a small series of patients and have little predictive power. Owing to their diverse methods and small sample sizes, none of these reports makes a strong case for an association between gluten and neuropsychiatric disorders.

What was missing was a major study conducted in a renowned institution involving large numbers of patients. In 2004, prompted by these reports, the U.S. National Institute of Mental Health (NIMH) launched a large-scale 5-year trial titled, "Diet and Behavior in Young

Children with Autism." Which investigated potential therapeutic benefits of a gluten and casein free diet in children with autism. As of January 2013, the study has been completed, but no publications resulting from the clinical trial have been released, yet the NIMH's trial shows how important this link may be.

If studies demonstrate beneficial effects of a gluten and casein free diet in children with autism, future trials could investigate such dietary effects in schizophrenia and ADHD. At present, as there are no negative side effects to being on a gluten-free diet, individuals suffering from one of these conditions may find that eliminating gluten has profound, long lasting benefits, especially if they are experiencing gastrointestinal symptoms.

Gluten Intolerance and Autism

Autism can include a wide variety of behaviors and characteristics, so professionals prefer the phrase autism spectrum disorder (ASD), which is more inclusive, and suggests a broad spectrum of neurological–developmental disorders that can occur in children with autism. Some children may display mild symptoms; but in others the disorder is more severe. We'll use autism here to refer to this spectrum of presentations, including what the National Institutes of Health describe as "pervasive developmental disorders."

Pervasive developmental disorders (PDD) is a broad category of conditions characterized by delays in development of communication and social skills. Autism is the most well known and best-studied of these disorders. Additional types of PDD include Asperger's syndrome and childhood disintegrative disorder.

Autism is characterized by impairments in verbal and nonverbal communication and in social interaction, as well as by restricted and repetitive stereotypical behaviors. Recently, the number of children affected by autistic disorders has risen. Its prevalence has increased dramatically within the last 20 years. The Centers for Disease Control and Prevention currently reports that approximately 1 in 68 children (14.7 per 1000 8-yearolds) were identified with autism spectrum disorder in a 2010 study. This estimate is 60% higher than that reported in 2006 (1 in 110).

Although the specific causes of autism are unknown, decades of research suggest that autism is associated with a complex set of environmental, genetic, neurological, and immunological factors. It is likely that each of these elements contributes to the development of autism in an individual, and each factor interacts with the others, but, preliminary evidence suggests that gluten may play an important role in the development of this disorder.

Immunological Response

What is the link between gluten intolerance and autism? In predisposed individuals, gluten intolerance causes certain immunological cells to produce biochemicals known as cytokines which perpetuate and extend an immunological reaction to a foreign protein such as gluten. Additionally cytokines can affect many behaviors, including social interactions, sleep, mood, appetite, and exploration.

Cytokines and other proinflammatory molecules have been found in increased concentrations in some children with autism, suggesting similarities in the processes that cause gluten intolerance and those related to autism. Also, high concentrations of specific autoantibodies against gluten are present in some children with autism, further suggesting a close relationship between gluten intolerance and autism.

Successful neurological development depends on a normally functioning immune response. Reports in the scientific literature point to abnormal or poorly regulated immune responses in children with autism. In some cases, autoimmune-type responses play a role in the development or maintenance of autism. The complex interactive relationship between the immune system and nervous system is well known, and immune system dysregulation can negatively impact nervous system structures. Subsequent changes in neurological functioning can lead to behaviors typical of autism.

In susceptible children, immune system antibodies created in response to gluten can cause a cascading immune response. Children with autism suffer gastrointestinal problems at a much higher rate than do other children. Symptoms include diarrhea, constipation, colic, abdominal pain, and gastroesophageal reflux. Studies report chronic gastrointestinal problems in children with autism at rates ranging from 17 to 24%. One study evaluated autistic children and control groups matched for age, sex, and ethnicity with 50 children in each group. Seventy percent of autistic children had gastrointestinal symptoms compared with 28% of children with typical development.

These gastrointestinal problems may be part of the overall autistic syndrome in selected children, and may also be part of the developmental pathology of autism. The digestive disorders may be related to gluten intolerance, and the cascading immunological effects of gluten intolerance may result in autism.

In some susceptible people, the cascading immune response provoked by gluten causes not only gastrointestinal problems, but also damage to certain areas of the brain, namely the cerebellum and the cerebral cortex, both of which are involved in autism. Cerebellar abnormalities are among the most consistent findings in people with autism.

Postmortem studies of autistic adults have demonstrated inflammatory cells in both the cerebral cortex and cerebellum, as well as autoantibodies to glial cells which are primary constituents of the brain. Glial cells provide support and protection for nerve cells and are the most abundant cell in the central nerve system. Autoantibodies to glial cells result in their death and breakdown as well as loss of function of the involved portion of the brain. Such an inflammatory/immune response to one's own neurological tissues can result from an overall hyperactivation of the immune system owing to the original immunological response to gluten.

A 2013 study utilizing 28 biopsy registries in Sweden demonstrated an increased risk of autism in individuals with positive celiac disease laboratory test results, confirming a strong association between autism and the presence of antibodies to gluten.

The Exorphin Connection

Most of us are familiar with endorphins, naturally occurring opiate-like biochemicals produced by specialized regions of our brain in response to vigorous exercise. These opioids are natural painkillers that create a sense of well-being. The commonly experienced "runner's high" results from an influx of endorphins and is associated with a heightened sense of self-esteem and increased creativity and productivity.

The "endo" prefix means these opioid proteins originate inside the body. A similar class of compounds found in substances derived from outside the body called exorphins were discovered approximately 30 years ago, and have been identified in samples of digested gluten and digested casein. Exorphins are absorbed from the digestive tract into the circulation and are able to cross the blood–brain barrier and affect the central nervous system.

Exorphins can play a role in causing the behavioral features of autism. Opioid proteins help regulate the development of the central nervous system, affecting the location, concentrations, and functions of specific nerve cells, so concentrations of opioids need to be tightly controlled. Excess amounts due to the presence of gluten-related exorphins may have a detrimental effect on brain development and behavior. Possible defects include abnormal locations and numbers of critically important nerve cells, as well as alterations in their functioning. In selected circumstances, autism can result from abnormal levels of exorphins derived from dietary gluten. The exorphin connection is a likely component of the complex relationship between gluten and autism.

Gluten-Free Diet and Improvement in Autistic Behavior

The presence of similar chronic gastrointestinal symptoms, including diarrhea, constipation, and abdominal pain in patients with gluten intolerance and in autistic children further strengthens the relationship between the diseases. Laboratory studies demonstrate additional findings in both disorders, including increased gastrointestinal permeability. Parents often report improvement of gastrointestinal symptoms and autistic behaviors after the child begins a strict gluten-free diet, suggesting a causal relationship with gluten.

For more than 25 years, reports in the scientific literature have described improvement in autistic behaviors following the adoption of gluten-free diets. Reports on a series of patients as well as open trials, both non-randomized and non-blinded, describe improvement across a range of behaviors, including:

- Communication skills
- Focusing
- Language use and comprehension

- Motor and sensory skills
- Sleep
- Social interaction

In addition, patients experienced a reduction in gastrointestinal symptoms and hyperactivity.

A comprehensive review tallying all available data in a meta-analysis demonstrated behavioral improvement in 66% of 2,561 children with autism following initiation of a gluten-free diet. These statistics suggest that if you have an autistic child, a gluten-free diet has a very strong likelihood of helping them improve.

Gluten Intolerance and Schizophrenia

Schizophrenia (from Greek roots meaning "split" and "mind") is a common mental disorder affecting almost 1% of the world's population and is one of the top ten causes of disability worldwide. Much research has been done on the genetic and environmental causes of this psychiatric disorder. As with autism, a strong connection between gluten intolerance and schizophrenia is suggested by a critical segment of this research.

Approximately 50 years ago, research suggested that celiac disease had numerous genes in common with schizophrenia. A clinical trial conducted at a Veterans Administration hospital, studied the effects of cereal-free and high-cereal diets on a group of 115 schizophrenic patients. Those randomly assigned to the cereal-free group were discharged from the hospital twice as fast as the high-cereal group. In a 1976 study of 14 schizophrenic patients, symptoms improved on average with a cereal-free diet, worsened when wheat products were added, and improved again when wheat was removed. Later, in the 1980s, population studies showed that schizophrenia was rare in cultures that consumed little or no grain. When wheat and barley were introduced into the diet, schizophrenia became common.

A well-known case study reported in the Journal of Internal Medicine in 1997 described the disappearance of psychiatric symptoms in a 33-year-old patient with schizophrenia following initiation of a gluten-free diet. Psychiatric symptoms improved after a few days. The patient had been malnourished, weighing only 85 pounds, but gluten intolerance and celiac disease often lead to chronic inflammation of the small intestine causing malabsorption syndrome, leading to malnutrition. After six months on the gluten-free diet the patient weighed 110 pounds, representing steady restoration of normal digestion. Of additional interest were computed tomography (CT) scans that had previously shown evidence of circulatory abnormalities in the patient's cerebral cortex associated with schizophrenia. A new CT scan, performed six months after the patient began the gluten-free diet, demonstrated that these abnormalities had completely resolved. The patient's anti-psychotic medications were discontinued at the time of her six-month follow-up, and she remained asymptomatic at a one-year follow-up.

A case report published in 2009 described a 70-year-old woman who received a diagnosis of schizophrenia at age 17. She experienced daily auditory and visual hallucinations, including hearing voices and seeing skeletons. She had been hospitalized at least five times in the prior six years for increasing psychotic symptoms and suicide attempts. Previously she had taken a range of anti-psychotic medications and was now instructed to follow a low-carbohydrate diet containing no grains. She returned for evaluation after seven days and reported that she no longer heard voices or saw skeletons. The patient continued her new diet for 12 months and had no recurrence of sensory hallucinations. The authors of the report concluded that medical treatment for schizophrenics could be augmented with a gluten-free diet with likely benefit.

The common link in these studies is gluten intolerance. Although the mechanisms are not completely understood, gluten may act as an environmental trigger for schizophrenia in genetically susceptible individuals. A population-based study conducted in Denmark, published in the British Medical Journal in 2004, reported an increased risk of developing schizophrenia in persons with a history of celiac disease. Important research focuses on the relationship between gluten intolerance and neuropsychiatric conditions such as schizophrenia.

The Exorphin Connection in Schizophrenia

Exorphins derived from dietary gluten may be implicated in the development of autism. In addition, they have been shown to affect other aspects of neuropsychiatric behavior and cause alterations in levels of neurotransmitters such as dopamine. Increased dopamine activity in the brain is hypothesized as a primary cause of the symptoms of schizophrenia.

The Genetic Connection

Research has clarified the genetic link between schizophrenia and gluten intolerance. A 2005 article published in Medical Hypotheses suggested that two genes related to celiac disease may work together to cause schizophrenia. Several studies published in Nature Genetics have reported a genetic marker for celiac disease located adjacent to a genetic marker for schizophrenia. A 2003 report in the American Journal of Human Genetics described chromosomal regions implicated in susceptibility to celiac disease that overlap chromosomal regions potentially related to susceptibility to schizophrenia.

These genetic relationships can result in altered physiology in susceptible individuals. In one proposed mechanism, the presence of specific genes leads to increased permeability of the small intestine and the blood–brain barrier. As a result, exorphins produced by digestion of gluten diffuse more readily into the circulation and transported more easily into central nervous system structures than is the case in other individuals. Such increased permeability leads to the development of celiac disease and schizophrenia.

As discussed in Chapter One, symptoms of gluten intolerance and celiac disease are caused by immune system reactions to dietary gluten. The enzyme tissue transglutaminase (tTG), found in cells located in the inner lining of the small intestine is a key component in this immune process. It's interesting to note that levels of circulating antibodies to gluten are significantly higher in patients with schizophrenia than in control subjects. Autoantibodies to tissue transglutaminase (found in those with gluten intolerance and celiac disease) cross-react with central nervous system structures, specifically with Purkinje cells (specialized neurons located in the cerebellum). As a result of such cross-targeting by autoantibodies to tTG, normally large Purkinje cells are significantly smaller in patients with schizophrenia. This pathology may be implicated in the development of schizophrenia.

Gluten Intolerance and Attention Deficit Hyperactivity Disorder

ADHD is the most commonly diagnosed behavioral disorder in children. The National Institute of Mental Health estimates that 9% of children between ages 13 and 18 are affected by it. The Centers for Disease Control and Prevention reports that in 2011, 11% of U.S. children between the ages of 4 and 17, (6.4 million children) had received a diagnosis of ADHD. The principal characteristics of ADHD include inability to pay attention, hyperactivity, and impulsive behaviors, but it may be difficult to diagnose as many children without ADHD demonstrate these characteristics in various combinations, at different intervals, and at varying levels of intensity. ADHD may be more accurately diagnosed when inattention, impulsiveness, and hyperactivity begin to affect behavior at home, performance at school, and interactions with other children. A diagnosis of ADHD requires the behaviors be of a degree inappropriate for others of comparable age.

Numerous studies have noted an association between celiac disease and neurological disorders such as ADHD, chronic headaches, and developmental delay. A study conducted in Israel in 2003 found that patients with celiac disease were much more likely to develop neurological disorders (51.4%) compared to control subjects (19.9%). ADHD is found in children and adults with celiac disease at a much higher frequency than in the general population. In the Israeli study, approximately 20% of the 111 patients with celiac disease also had ADHD and related learning disabilities. In some people, the only symptoms of gluten sensitivity may be neurological, such as those found in ADHD. Symptoms of celiac disease can appear years after the onset of ADHD or other neurological disorders.

A gluten-free diet is often effective in reducing or eliminating ADHD symptoms. A study conducted in the Netherlands in 2002 found behavioral improvement in 25 of 40 (62%) children who met the DMS-IV criteria for ADHD and who followed a gluten-free diet.

The Conners Comprehensive Behavior Rating Scale and the ADHD Rating Scale were utilized to evaluate ADHD status. A follow-up study performed in 2008 found that a gluten free diet resulted in significant improvement in 73% of children with ADHD (11 of 15 children) compared to 0% in the control group (0 of 12 children). All of these studies stress the importance of large-scale clinical trials, but the evidence to date is sufficiently clear to go forward with at-home practical implementation. There are no negative side effects of a gluten-free diet and the improvements documented in the research suggest your child may benefit greatly with this therapeutic approach. Your child's ability to learn and engage in fulfilling and enriching friendships, and their ability to contribute to the welfare of their family will grow and develop as the burdens of ADHD recede and dissolve. A gluten-free diet is an important part of the solution.

Additional Gluten-Related Neurological Disorders:
— Gluten Ataxia

Ataxia is a neurological condition involving significant lack of muscular coordination. Cerebellar ataxia is caused by disrupted neurological activity in the cerebellum. When your doctor asks you to close your eyes and touch your nose with the tip of your index finger, she's testing cerebellar coordination. Likewise, when a police officer or state trooper asks a person to step out of the car and walk a straight line, heel-to-toe, she's testing cerebellar coordination—which can be disrupted by excessive alcohol intake.

Peripheral neuropathy is a disorder of the long nerves in your body. For example, the sciatic nerve in your leg or the median nerve in your forearm. The most common symptoms are pain and numbness.

As we've discussed, gluten intolerance has been linked with a number of complex neuropsychiatric disorders including autism, schizophrenia, and ADHD. It is also associated with purely neurological entities including ataxia and peripheral neuropathy. Gluten ataxia, first described in 1966, usually affects the gait and is frequently accompanied by peripheral neuropathy. Not every case of ataxia is caused by gluten, but the association with gluten is a diagnosis of exclusion when other alternative explanations have been considered and eliminated.

> **Idiopathic sporadic ataxia** refers to irregularly occurring ataxia of unknown origin. Typical causes of ataxia include multiple sclerosis, stroke, brain tumor, vitamin B_{12} deficiency, and alcohol intoxication. In idiopathic ataxia, the patient demonstrates loss of muscular coordination, but a cause of the disorder is not found. Gluten intolerance and celiac disease may be a cause of such ataxia. Research has shown that up to 60% of patients with gluten ataxia have cerebellar atrophy.

A 2008 review published in *The Cerebellum* suggests gluten ataxia as a common cause of idiopathic sporadic ataxia. Anti-gluten antibodies are frequently found in higher proportions in such cases than in the general population. Peripheral neuropathy has also been found in up to 49% of patients with celiac disease.

Earlier we mentioned that antibodies to gluten have been shown to cross-react with Purkinje cells. Patchy loss of these specialized neurons has been demonstrated in postmortem studies of patients with gluten ataxia.

Studies have shown that a gluten-free diet has consistently improved symptoms of idiopathic sporadic ataxia. One systematic study using a control group reported on 43 patients with gluten ataxia. Twenty-six patients began a gluten-free diet and achieved significant improvement in neurological testing and overall clinical impressions. The study concluded that a gluten-free diet appeared to be an effective treatment for gluten ataxia.

It is widely accepted that patients with ataxia of unknown cause should be screened for gluten intolerance and celiac disease.

The Celiac "Iceberg" and the Importance of Screening

The World Health Organization (WHO) criteria for widespread screening of specific diseases include:

- A suitable screening test or examination should be available
- The disease process should be sufficiently understood
- An accepted method of treatment should be available for patients with the disease
- Treatment begun at an earlier stage of the disease should be more beneficial than treatment started later on

- Costs of screening should be balanced against overall costs of treatment

Celiac disease meets the WHO requirements for widespread screening and is related to immunological abnormalities. There is an effective treatment program — a lifetime gluten-free diet. Community-based screening for celiac disease would enable definitive treatment for many individuals who have been suffering without hope of relief. The scientific literature consistently reports that celiac disease is significantly underdiagnosed and underreported. This fact has been termed the celiac "iceberg" as those patients who have received a diagnosis of gluten intolerance or celiac disease represent only a fraction of those actually affected.

Celiac disease screening would be of particular importance to individuals with schizophrenia. As we've seen, not only is celiac disease found frequently in patients with schizophrenia, it is also a likely causative factor in its development. Physicians need to be aware of this relationship and families need to ensure that loved ones with schizophrenia are screened for celiac disease.

How to Achieve Meaningful Change

Does every child, teenager, or young adult with autism, schizophrenia, or ADHD also have gluten intolerance? No, but young people with one of these neuropsychiatric disorders have a much greater likelihood of being gluten intolerant than a young person in the general population. A great deal of documentation in peer-reviewed literature suggests that gluten intolerance is linked to these disorders and a gluten-free diet may significantly improve a young person's symptoms.

Young people with one of these conditions undergo daily stress that may be severe. Their parents, siblings, and close relatives experience similarly intense day-to-day stress. The road for these young persons and their families is long, hard, and seems to extend endlessly into a compromised future of medication, doctor's visits, and unfulfilled aspirations. Benefits from a gluten-free diet may seem too good to be true. How could something so simple and prosaic be of any use, when the "best" specialists don't have effective solutions?

We've presented much scientific evidence pointing toward the effectiveness of a gluten-free diet in subsets of young people with these disorders. If a particular individual is susceptible to gluten intolerance, a gluten-free diet will make a big difference. Choosing to institute such a diet can provide substantial, ongoing benefits. There is no downside to this course of action.

You won't be wasting time by trying one medication versus another. Your child may remain on their medications while instituting a gluten-free diet and if symptoms improve, there may be an opportunity to reduce the dosage or eliminate the medications which would be a significant result.

There are no negative side effects of a gluten-free diet. Wheat, barley, and rye are not critical components of anyone's diet, but wheat, barley, and rye may be a real problem for your child.

Going Gluten-Free

Once you've decided that a gluten-free diet may be right for your child, it's important to begin this new lifestyle effectively. The first thing to remember is that you don't want you and your child to struggle. You want the implementation of a gluten-free diet to be a positive change rather than a burden. It's best to think of your new way of living as a choice, as opposed to something you have to do.

Remember, be kind to yourself and your family members as you take action. It will be much easier if the entire household goes gluten-free than one family member doing it alone, which requires separate foods, dishware, toasters, toaster ovens, and food preparation areas. Also, it's not necessary to do everything at once in a revolutionary kitchen-and-refrigerator coup-d'état. Instead, take small graduated steps that get the job done while minimizing emotional stress.

Use your first two weeks to remove all gluten-containing foods from your refrigerator, kitchen cabinets, and pantry. Make sure to remove all gluten-containing household supplies from your cellar, attic, and bathroom. Certain toothpastes, sunscreens, laundry detergents, soaps, shampoos, and lotions contain gluten.

What do these products have to do with gluten intolerance? Dermatitis herpetiformis, an itchy, burning, painful skin eruption, may be a symptom of a child's immune response to gluten. Other gluten-related skin disorders include hives and rashes. Gluten in these household products can remain on your child's hands and ingested through contact with the lips or mouth. Some over-the-counter medications may also contain gluten that is used in manufacturing and processing.

It may sound like a lot of trouble, but the one-time inconvenience of tossing all these products in the trash may be outweighed by the gratifying improvements in your child's behaviors.

Gluten-free foods and household products are available in supermarkets, natural food markets, and many well-established online stores. Numerous well-known national brands supply a diverse array of gluten-free products to a variety of commercial outlets and many companies have earned gluten-free certification from either the Celiac Support Association or the Gluten Intolerance Group. Their websites list the companies who have met the gluten-free standards. (csaceliacs.org and gfco.org)

Once you've restocked, gradually introduce gluten-free dishes at breakfast, lunch, and dinner. Fresh meat, fish, and poultry are always gluten-free, as are fresh fruits and vegetables, so there is always plenty of variety. What you're specifically adding to your family's diet is gluten-free versions of cereals, pancakes, waffles, breads, muffins, pastas, sauces, desserts, and snacks.

It's important that your child remain gluten-free at school as well as home. You can prepare a plastic tub of gluten-free supplies such as markers, paints, crayons, and soap and request that the tub remain in the classroom with the other supplies. It's a good idea to alert the teacher to your child's health concerns. Ideally, the teacher will become your ally and help your child remain fully engaged in class activities while maintaining a gluten-free status.

The Parent Advantage

Parents have a huge advantage relative to physicians when it comes to prescribing a gluten-free diet for a child with autism or one of the other disorders we've discussed. Unlike doctors, parents don't have to wait for publication of randomized, double-blind peer-reviewed studies proving that implementation of a gluten-free diet leads to improvement in autistic behaviors. As we've seen, the scientific literature reported that a gluten-free diet led to improvement in two-thirds of 2,561 autistic children.

Your doctor may be hesitant to recommend this course of action as results of large trials aren't currently available. On the other hand, your doctor may be unfamiliar with the benefits of a gluten-free diet. In either case, the possibilities of symptomatic improvement and benefit to your child as well as the absence of any risk are well worth your time and effort.

If after 3-4 months, on a gluten-free diet, behavior is improved, your child and family have created a new world in which to live where old struggles and challenges will recede. There will be new ones, but your family will have gained a sense of empowerment to meet them effectively.

Gluten Intolerance and Endocrine Disorders: Diabetes, Thyroid Disease, and Addison's Disease

The Farmer's Daughter

"I was a real farm girl," said Martha Brolin. "We did the sunup to sundown thing." She paused, her blue eyes sparkling. "Kind of the opposite of vampires, if you know what I mean." The light in her eyes dims. "Bet if I were a vampire, I wouldn't have had to go through what I did, though I guess there'd be some not-so-pleasant disadvantages."

In the 1980s, Martha's active imagination was honed by the discipline of her Nebraska childhood. Baling hay and cleaning chicken coops can have a remarkable effect on a young mind, and she had a strong sense of how lucky she was. A pint-sized hybrid of the Greek goddesses Artemis and Demeter, Martha rose with the sun and launched herself daily on a poetical journey. At dinner she regaled her brothers, sisters, and guests with convoluted tales of her adventures of the last 24 hours. Her parents took the hint and presented her with a black leather journal for her ninth birthday so she recorded each day's events along with snippets of local news and wrote verse as well as stories. She soon needed her second and her third journal.

The editor of the local paper encouraged Martha to submit pieces to the Sunday edition and by the time she started high school, she won several writing contests and became an occasional contributor to the Omaha World-Herald and Nebraska Journal Star. Additionally, the faculty adviser for her school weekly had promised her a regular column, but without warning, at age 15, Martha's health fell apart. She fainted in geometry class while working out a proof on the whiteboard. The next day her classmates joked that the problem was too hard. Martha laughed with them, but fainted again later in the week in English class. "I can't blame this on Euclid," she told her mother. "I was in English class. We were reading Ivanhoe, not Wuthering Heights. Knights don't faint."

Despite her good humor and the efforts of various doctors, Martha's health got worse.

"When you grow up on a farm you're supposed to be robust," she said. "Plenty of sunshine, fresh air, fresh food, ruddy cheeks, and clear skin with an outdoor glow. The whole nine yards. Guess I fumbled on the tenth yard."

> **Epstein-Barr virus (EBV)** is a common herpesvirus. Most adults carry EBV as a dormant virus. However, under certain circumstances the virus can get reactivated. Symptoms of EBV reactivation include fatigue, headache, brain fog, muscle soreness, and fever.

Martha rarely missed classes throughout grade school and junior high. Now she found herself literally flat on her back, profoundly fatigued, and so weak it was difficult to get up when she wanted a glass of water. No one knew what was wrong. Her pediatrician ordered a series of blood tests, but everything came back normal. Infection with the Epstein-Barr virus was a popular diagnosis at the time, about 30 years ago, and her doctor decided Martha was infected with it. There's no specific treatment other than rest, so Martha's parents were told, "Just wait a bit. She'll get over it."

Absent from school for long stretches at a time, Martha gathered enough strength to go back to class for a few days, but soon grew so tired she had to stay home again. She cycled back and forth like this throughout that first autumn and the early part of winter. Her teachers allowed her to keep up with assignments and homework, but this wasn't how Martha thought high school should be. She missed her classmates and missed the social scene, then remarkably, she felt better and returned for the rest of the school year.

"Did you have mono?" a few girls giggled at lunch her first day back. Martha ignored them, knowing she might expect a lot worse.

Her status had been reduced to that of a "new kid." Despite the razzing, she was glad to be in class instead of lying around at home, and she made it through the first day, the first week, and the first month. She felt good and had perfect attendance the rest of the school year, but a few months later, in mid-September, her symptoms resurfaced and Martha missed most of the fall semester. She returned after New Year's and managed to stay in class for the rest of the year. During the summer she tried to enjoy herself, but dreaded another autumn season of misery.

When school started, she decided to tough it out no matter how she felt. Every day her mother asked how she was feeling, and every day Martha gritted her teeth and said, "Fine." She endured through sheer strength of character and force of will, but finally collapsed one morning in early October while waiting for the school bus. By this point Martha, her family, and her teachers knew the drill. She didn't even try to go back to school until Thanksgiving and returned to class full-time in January. Thankfully, high school graduation was approaching.

Martha admitted that she "was always kind of sick in school." Aware of her mysterious seasonal affliction she was concerned about getting a job after graduation, but she received many offers. Thanks to her outgoing personality and excellent grades, Martha accepted a position at the local branch of a national bank and was promoted consistently. Though she seemed to have left her health problems behind, Martha wasn't sanguine and as it turned out, she was right not to take too much for granted.

Shortly after receiving a promotion to the head of her department, Martha began experiencing mild forgetfulness, but didn't think anything was wrong. She was busy at work and had a lot of responsibility. Anyone could forget an appointment or a scheduled phone call, but a few weeks later she became disoriented and her muscle aches and joint pains returned.

Her aches and pains progressed to such an extent that she needed to leave work at 4:00 p.m. or earlier every day. Her manager was sympathetic and suggested installing a comfortable sofa in the staff break room, hoping to provide an opportunity for Martha to rest and relax so she could complete a full day at the bank. Martha hoped to avoid the same problems she experienced as a teenager, but despite her valiant efforts and the support of her co-workers, her symptoms worsened.

"I found I had a hard time getting out of bed," she said. Even when she made it to work, Martha had to lie down more frequently and her breaks became longer while her muscle and joint pains increased. She often felt nauseated and suffered headaches almost every day. When her disorientation became obvious a co-worker suggested she might have "cognitive dysfunction." Martha hadn't heard this term before and looked it up on the Internet where she encountered the more common term, "brain fog."

"That sounds right," she thought. "I'm forgetful, I have difficulty concentrating, and I get confused easily. What's wrong with me?" As sick as she'd been in high school, Martha had never really been scared, but now at 28, she was older and had to acknowledge she was actually frightened.

> The **adrenal glands** are small, pyramid-shaped structures located on top of each kidney. In adrenal insufficiency, these glands are not manufacturing sufficient amounts of steroid hormones, including cortisol. Adrenal insufficiency may be caused by an autoimmune disease of the glands themselves, severe infection, or a congenital condition.

Friends recommended doctors and after a few medical misfires, Martha found an endocrinologist who possessed an effective combination of skill and expertise who diagnosed her diverse symptoms as autoimmune polyglandular syndrome type 2 (Schmidt syndrome), which includes adrenal insufficiency and an additional endocrine disorder which is typically either hypothyroidism or type 1 diabetes. In Martha's case, adrenal insufficiency was a result of the autoimmune disorder Addison's disease. Martha's second medical problem was Hashimoto's thyroiditis, a cause of hypothyroidism.

All of her symptoms could be attributed to the combination of adrenal and thyroid gland diseases. Addison's disease was causing autoimmune destruction of her adrenal glands, leading to muscle and joint pain, weakness, nausea, fatigue, and disorientation owing to loss of sodium and potassium electrolytes. Hashimoto's thyroiditis was causing autoimmune destruction of her thyroid gland, leading to muscle weakness, fatigue, memory loss, headaches, and irregular heart rhythm. Her endocrine system was being attacked from two directions and she was lucky to have gotten an accurate diagnosis.

When Martha's doctor placed her on hydrocortisone and Synthroid to replace the missing corticosteroid and thyroid hormones she felt better and returned to the bank full-time, but there were more medical difficulties ahead.

Three years later in 2008, Martha and her family moved to Southern California and in 2009 she again became fatigued and experienced abdominal pain and diarrhea. Her muscle pains returned on a more severe basis, and she developed severe bone pain. In great distress, Martha didn't know where to get good advice. Her endocrinologist was back in Nebraska, and Martha wasn't confident she could find a suitable replacement.

Both she and her husband made inquiries which directed Martha to our clinic. After her initial assessment, we told Martha that her new abdominal pain and diarrhea, as well as the muscle and bone pain were caused by celiac disease. Her lab tests indicated that she carried genes for DQ2 and DQ8, genetic markers for gluten intolerance. She was told how celiac disease affects many body systems, owing to malabsorption of nutrients as well as a potentially widespread immunological response. Martha began a gluten-free diet under our guidance and her health improved within a week. The new diet made a big difference and Martha felt better for several years.

In 2013, Martha noticed she had to urinate more frequently and over the next two months this worsened until she had to urinate every 20 minutes. In addition, she was fainting several times a week and worried that she wouldn't be able to drive safely. Eventually she was urinating every 10 minutes and became severely dehydrated. She also experienced severe chest pains and felt as if she was having a heart attack, so an ambulance was called.

The next day in the coronary care unit a resident shared with Martha that she "had almost coded." Her electrolytes were depleted and her coronary episode was the result. Her potassium and sodium levels were extremely low owing to her frequent urination, which was caused by diabetes insipidus (water diabetes).

For Martha and her physicians, diabetes insipidus could represent an unwelcome extension of autoimmune polyglandular disorder type 2. Diabetes insipidus results from damage to the pituitary gland which can be caused by the same autoimmune processes that damaged Martha's adrenal and thyroid glands. Although this is uncommon, Martha was genetically predisposed to such autoimmune disorders. Her doctors started her on the hormone vasopressin which she lacked owing to her pituitary problem.

Martha has had a difficult medical journey. Some days are better than others, but she is improving. She can drive and usually gets out of bed in the morning without trouble. Occasionally she needs hospitalization to receive intravenous infusions of electrolytes (vasopressin causes sodium and potassium loss), but she accepts this as a small price for being reasonably healthy.

Martha described the critical importance of a strict gluten-free diet and finding a rheumatologist, internist, or endocrinologist who understands gluten intolerance and celiac disease. "If there's anyone I can help get through these kinds of problems," she said, "I'm happy to provide support. I know I have some weird stuff, and I'm glad to help."

She also mentioned the importance of knowing your family history. "My mother has had celiac disease for 25 years," she said. "One of my sisters has type 1 diabetes and all kinds of arthritis. My other sister has hip problems and type 1 diabetes. My niece has celiac disease. My father has thyroid problems and type 1 diabetes. I learned I inherited a lot of my health problems from my Mom and Dad."

Gluten Intolerance and Type 1 Diabetes

Insulin is a hormone produced by specialized cells in the pancreas. It has many functions, including causing muscle and liver cells to absorb glucose from the bloodstream. Without sufficient insulin or a normal physiological response to insulin, blood glucose levels remain high.

Diabetes is a group of diseases caused by impaired insulin production, defective insulin action, or both. The key clinical finding in diabetes is elevated blood glucose (sugar) levels, caused by problems with the hormone insulin. Serious pathologies are associated with diabetes, owing to glucose-related damage to small blood vessels in organs such as the kidneys and eyes, and there is evidence of a link between this complex, debilitating disease and gluten intolerance.

In 2012, 29 million Americans, more than 9% of the population, had diabetes and it is the fifth leading cause of death in the United States. There were 1.7 million new cases in the United States in 2012 among people 20 years of age or older and in 2012 an estimated 86 million Americans aged 20 or older were pre-diabetic. Without effective preventive measures, such individuals are considered at risk of developing type 2 diabetes. These figures attest to the epidemic nature of diabetes in the United States, but this epidemic is not confined to Americans. Worldwide figures are comparable.

According to the WHO, the global prevalence of diabetes among adults older than age 18 is estimated to be 9% and worldwide diabetes is projected to be the seventh leading cause of death by 2030. Not only are more new cases of type 1 diabetes appearing every year, but earlier age of onset is apparent. Type 1 diabetes is progressively appearing in younger children. Overall, the annual number of new cases was estimated to be approximately 40% higher in 2010 than in 1997.

Type 1 diabetes, known as juvenile-onset diabetes involves impaired glucose production. Type 2 diabetes, previously known as adult-onset diabetes, has been increasing in frequency in younger people for many years and is related to defective insulin action. This lack of response is known as insulin resistance.

Diabetes is a serious problem owing to the effects of chronically elevated blood glucose levels. High concentrations of glucose molecules cause deposits in the walls of small blood vessels and small arteries become blocked which results in ongoing damage to tissues and organs. People with uncontrolled diabetes with blood glucose levels too high for too long may develop loss of vision, loss of circulation in their feet and legs, and kidney problems. Left untreated, such people may lose their sight, need to have a foot amputated, or suffer kidney failure which can lead to death.

Many people with diabetes have high cholesterol levels and elevated blood pressure that results from a number of factors, including blockage of small arteries caused by cholesterol deposits. Cardiovascular disease and diabetes are related disorders. Two of every three people with type 1 or type 2 diabetes will die of heart disease or stroke. In type 1 diabetes, the pancreas no longer makes insulin. Affected individuals require daily insulin injections for hormone replacement. Type 2 diabetes is characterized as a lifestyle disease caused by years of poor nutrition and lack of exercise. Muscle cells develop a tolerance to insulin owing to chronically elevated levels of serum glucose and severe daily fluctuations in insulin levels. Muscle cells become "insulin resistant" and no longer respond to the hormone. In these cases, blood glucose remains high and the person develops symptoms of diabetes.

Type 1 Diabetes, Autoimmunity, and Gluten Intolerance

> The **islets of Langerhans** are small "islands" of specialized hormone-producing cells located throughout the pancreas. The islets comprise approximately 1–2% of the mass of the pancreas. Pancreatic "beta cells" are islet cells that produce insulin.

In the last several decades, type 1 diabetes has been recognized as an autoimmune disorder. The first evidence for this relationship was based on the observation that type 1 diabetes was frequently found in the presence of other endocrine (hormone-producing) autoimmune diseases. Insulin is produced in the pancreas by specialized cells comprising the islets of Langerhans. In type 1 diabetes these specialized cells are destroyed by autoimmune inflammatory processes causing the ability to produce insulin to be permanently lost. Such autoimmunity suggests a relationship with other autoimmune disorders such as celiac disease. The association between celiac disease and type 1 diabetes was recognized more than 30 years ago and many studies have since demonstrated this relationship.

A 2001 study demonstrated that 27.4% of 197 patients with type 1 diabetes had two or more autoantibodies specific for type 1 diabetes, celiac disease, and autoimmune thyroid disease. In 150 healthy control subjects, 0% had such autoantibodies.

Studies have shown that celiac disease is present in 5% of patients (range, 1.4–16%) with type 1 diabetes. This prevalence is much higher than in the general population (1%). Similarly, 11% of patients with celiac disease were found to have diabetes-related autoantibodies. As a comparison, the prevalence of type 1 diabetes in the U.S. is 0.12%, so type 1 diabetes–related autoantibodies are found approximately 100 times more frequently in those with celiac disease.

What is responsible for this unusual and unexpected relationship?

Hereditary factors are usually cited when describing these associations and can lead to a tendency to develop autoimmune diseases. Prolonged exposure to gluten in susceptible individuals is also considered a contributing factor in the development of autoimmune diseases such as autoimmune thyroiditis, Addison's disease, and type 1 diabetes.

The genetic predisposition suggests that celiac disease runs in families. First-degree relatives, parents, siblings, and children of individuals with celiac disease have a ten-fold greater likelihood of developing the disease than others. If one identical twin is diagnosed with celiac disease, the chance of the other twin having it is 80%. The specific genetic similarity between celiac disease and diabetes involves human leukocyte antigens DQ2 and DQ8 (HLA DQ2 was discussed in Chapter Two). As in celiac disease, first-degree relatives of patients with type 1 diabetes have an increased prevalence of these HLA proteins.

Additionally, HLA DQ2 and DQ8 proteins are identified in other autoimmune diseases including Addison's disease, Hashimoto's thyroiditis, and autoimmune liver disease. The prevalence of celiac disease is increased in patients with these autoimmune conditions. One hypothesis suggests the chronic immune response in gluten intolerance and celiac disease "cross-reacts" with other normal proteins in the body, causing autoimmune reactions to endocrine glands such as the adrenal glands, thyroid, and liver. The result can be chronic endocrine autoimmune disease.

Benefits of a Gluten-Free Diet in Type 1 Diabetes

If the chronic immune reaction in celiac disease is related to the development of type 1 diabetes, a gluten-free diet may be helpful in diabetes treatment in its early stages and early detection of celiac disease can prevent the development of diabetes and other autoimmune diseases. One study evaluated adolescent patients recently diagnosed with celiac disease. Diabetes-related antibodies were found in 11 of 90 patients (11.1%). After 24 months of following a strict gluten-free diet, all 11 patients were free of diabetes-related antibodies. This result has important implications for diabetes prevention worldwide.

Researchers in the United Kingdom state that a gluten-free diet improves glycemic control in patients with type 1 diabetes. Improved glycemic control that maintains relatively normal levels of blood glucose helps minimize the problems associated with hyperglycemia and hypoglycemia.

Hypoglycemia or low blood sugar is a common problem in type 1 diabetes caused by taking too much insulin, certain medications, or eating a meal with too many simple sugars. Symptoms include dizziness, rapid heart rate, weakness, and anxiety. Without treatment hypoglycemia can cause fainting, seizures, and possibly diabetic coma.

Hyperglycemia or high blood sugar occurs when there is an excessive amount of glucose in the blood plasma. Chronic hyperglycemia can produce a wide variety of complications over a period of years, including kidney damage, neurological damage, cardiovascular damage, damage to the retina or damage to feet and legs.

A study in Denmark evaluated 25% of the Danish population. Researchers identified 303 adolescents with type 1 diabetes. Of these, 269 participated in the study and were examined for celiac disease. Thirty-three cases of celiac disease (12.3%) were found, representing the highest such prevalence in Europe. Diabetic patients with celiac disease had diminished height and weighed less compared to the rest of the group and diabetes began at a significantly younger age in those with celiac disease.

Celiac patients were started on a gluten-free diet. After 24 months, these young people had significant increases in height and weight and two patients had fewer episodes of hypoglycemia, suggesting a diabetes treatment effect caused by the gluten-free diet.

Early detection of celiac disease may reduce the occurrence of type 1 diabetes in children. In young children, abdominal swelling, gas, and diarrhea may suggest the presence of gluten intolerance and celiac disease. Toddlers with these conditions are shorter and weigh less. Such inhibited growth is known as failure to thrive. Any child persistently demonstrating any of these features should be evaluated for celiac disease. If gluten intolerance and celiac disease is discovered sooner rather than later, the development of autoimmune disorders such as type 1 diabetes can be prevented. Research shows that with a gluten-free diet, these children gain weight and grow taller. Their ability to thrive is restored. Removing gluten eliminates the immune mechanism causing the production of diabetes autoantibodies, and these autoantibodies disappear from the children's blood, proving that a gluten-free diet reduces the threat of diabetes in children with a genetic susceptibility.

Gluten Intolerance and Autoimmune Thyroiditis (Hashimoto's Disease and Graves' Disease)

The mechanism of autoimmune thyroiditis results in two types of disease. In Hashimoto's disease (chronic lymphocytic thyroiditis), anti-thyroid autoantibodies attack thyroid hormone–producing cells. The result is insufficient amounts of thyroid hormone, known as hypothyroidism. In Graves' disease, anti-thyroid autoantibodies attack specialized thyroid proteins. The result is a markedly enlarged thyroid gland (goiter) and overproduction of thyroid hormone, known as hyperthyroidism.

Hashimoto's disease is the most common cause of hypothyroidism in the United States affecting between 0.1 and 5% of all adults in Western countries and is most common in middle-aged women. Hashimoto's disease affects more than 1 million people in the United States. Symptoms include:

- Constipation
- Difficulty concentrating (brain fog)
- Dry skin
- Hair loss
- Joint stiffness
- Swelling of the face
- Weight gain

Some individuals may be symptom-free and with treatment, the prognosis in Hashimoto's disease is very good.
Graves' disease affects more than 1 million people in the United States and is most common in women.

Symptoms include:

- Anxiety
- Bulging eyes (exophthalmos)
- Fatigue
- Increased sweating
- Muscle weakness
- Rapid heart rate
- Tremor
- Shortness of breath
- Weight loss

Left untreated, complications of Graves' disease include cardiovascular disease and osteoporosis.

As with type 1 diabetes, autoimmune thyroiditis may be associated with gluten intolerance and celiac disease. One study found that 14.4% of patients with celiac disease had anti-thyroid autoantibodies in their bloodstream which appeared to be related to dietary gluten. A gluten-free diet resulted in the disappearance of these autoantibodies on follow-up testing after 24 months in 85% of patients. These researchers proposed that starting a gluten-free diet as soon as possible in children with celiac disease might help prevent development of additional autoimmune diseases.

A study reviewing evidence on autoimmune disorders showed that approximately 10–15% of patients with celiac disease have autoimmune thyroid disease, presenting as either hypo or hyperthyroidism. This frequency is at least 10-fold higher than in the general population. Conversely, approximately 4% of those with autoimmune thyroid disorders have celiac disease, representing a four-fold increase compared to the overall population. A 2005 study performed in the United Kingdom evaluated 111 patients with Graves' disease. Of these, five were shown to have celiac disease (4.5%). A 1999 study done in Italy found celiac disease in four of 92 patients with autoimmune thyroid disease (4.3%). Additional research demonstrates that as many as 43% of patients with Hashimoto's disease had immunologic markers typical of celiac disease.

In another study performed in Italy, six of 172 patients (3.4%) with autoimmune thyroiditis had celiac disease autoantibodies in their bloodstream. This compared with ten such individuals (0.25%) in a sample of 4,000 random blood donors. The authors concluded there is a close relationship between celiac disease and other autoimmune diseases and recommend screening for celiac disease in patients with other autoimmune disorders to limit future risk and possibly reduce symptoms.

In terms of accuracy of diagnosis, it is possible to mistake symptoms of thyroid disorders for those of gluten intolerance and celiac disease. Fatigue, muscle weakness, constipation, joint pain, and brain fog are common symptoms in both celiac disease and autoimmune thyroid disease, but gluten intolerance and celiac disease can demonstrate minimal or no symptoms at a certain point in the patient's history. Screening for celiac disease in all individuals at risk for autoimmune thyroid disease would be an important and beneficial public health measure. Patients with gluten intolerance and celiac disease should be tested for abnormalities in thyroid function. The benefits of early diagnosis are considerable in all these conditions.

There have been several reports of improvement in symptoms of autoimmune thyroiditis following diagnosis and treatment of co-existing celiac disease. Untreated celiac disease can perpetuate co-existing autoimmune disorders such as autoimmune thyroiditis, probably resulting from the ongoing autoimmune response to gluten. Researchers in Canada reported on a patient with autoimmune thyroid disease who received thyroid hormone replacement therapy. The patient wasn't improving and lab tests showed she wasn't absorbing the hormone properly from her gastrointestinal tract. Further examination led to a diagnosis of celiac disease, which caused the malabsorption. The authors of the report stressed the importance of screening for multiple endocrine diseases in patients with autoimmune endocrine disorders.

A similar case was reported in a 2009 paper where a patient with Graves' disease took several medications to control her symptoms. She was also being evaluated for iron-deficiency anemia. Laboratory tests indicated that celiac disease was the cause of her anemia. Two months after starting a gluten-free diet the patient was no longer anemic and the symptoms of Graves' disease improved. She was able to discontinue her anti-thyroid medications and remained symptom-free when she was examined one year later. The authors stressed the important finding that early diagnosis of celiac disease can reverse some thyroid abnormalities.

Another study demonstrated full recovery of autoimmune thyroid disease following initiation of a gluten-free diet. More research involving larger groups needs to be done to further evaluate the benefits of a gluten-free diet in autoimmune thyroiditis.

Combined Autoimmune Disorders—Autoimmune Thyroiditis, Type 1 Diabetes, and Celiac Disease

Multiple autoimmune disorders often occur in the same patient. A 2007 study investigated 370 children and adolescents with type 1 diabetes which had been present in these young people for an average of seven years. Patients were evaluated for the presence of anti-thyroid autoantibodies and autoantibodies characteristic of celiac disease. Anti-thyroid autoantibodies were found in 42 patients (11.4%; 10 times higher than in the general population) and celiac disease autoantibodies were found in nine patients (3.2%; three times higher than in the general population).

The frequency of anti-thyroid autoantibodies increased as the young people got older. Anti-thyroid autoantibodies were present in 28% of girls and 12% of boys by the time they reached 18 years of age. This phenomenon is similar to the increasing prevalence of type 1 diabetes found in children with celiac disease as they get older.

Gluten Intolerance, Celiac Disease, and Addison's Disease

Cortisol is a glucocorticoid hormone that helps the body convert food into energy, helps restore metabolic balance after a stress response, and is part of the immune system's inflammatory response.

Aldosterone is a mineralocorticoid hormone that maintains the body's balance of sodium and potassium and helps maintain blood pressure at normal levels.

Addison's disease is an autoimmune disorder affecting the adrenal glands. In Addison's disease the cells of the outer layer of the adrenal glands known as the adrenal cortex are destroyed and the body's ability to produce adrenal cortical hormones is progressively lost. These hormones include cortisol and aldosterone.

Addison's disease is rare in the general population (less than 2 cases per 10,000 persons; less than 0.02%), but can be fatal if undiagnosed and untreated. Addison's disease causes nausea, vomiting, abdominal pain, weight loss, fatigue, muscle weakness, headache, and mood swings. It also causes darkening of the skin. A severely ill person can faint, have a fever, undergo convulsions, and go into a hypoglycemic coma.

Chronic Addison's disease is often difficult to diagnose. Affected persons experience fatigue, generalized weakness, and overall discomfort and malaise. They just don't feel well. Additional symptoms can include abdominal cramps and weight loss. Many other disorders feature the same set of symptoms, making the specific diagnosis difficult. As Addison's disease is rare in the general population, many doctors and internists may not consider it as a possible cause of their patient's condition. As with gluten intolerance and celiac disease, physicians' index of suspicion needs to be raised.

Although Addison's disease is rare, there is an increased risk in people with gluten intolerance and celiac disease. A 2007 study conducted in Sweden evaluated the medical records of 15,439 persons with a diagnosis of celiac disease. The study included a control group of 70,095 persons. These researchers found 39 cases of Addison's disease in the group with celiac disease (0.25%) and 19 cases of Addison's disease in the control group (0.02%). Those with celiac disease had a ten-fold greater risk of developing Addison's disease compared to the general population.

From the reverse perspective, a smaller study done in 2001 in Ireland screened 41 patients with Addison's disease. Of these, 5 had celiac disease (12.2%). This prevalence of celiac disease is 12 times higher than in the general population.

This increased risk is related to certain genetic features that are common to both diseases. As with type 1 diabetes, autoimmune thyroid diseases, gluten intolerance, and celiac disease, persons with Addison's disease commonly have the genetic traits of HLA DQ2 and DQ8 proteins.

Screening and Diagnosis

Screening makes great sense for populations at risk for serious diseases. The main question is at what level of risk does screening begin? Many recent large studies have shown that screening for prostate cancer may not provide significant health value, but for populations who already have one disorder, screening for serious related conditions should be standard procedure.

There are several obstacles to diagnosing gluten intolerance and celiac disease. First, these disorders may not cause any symptoms until there has been a fair amount of progression. Those with an increased risk (first-degree relatives parents, siblings, and children) who have gluten intolerance should be screened for these conditions and individuals with any of the conditions we've been discussing should be screened for gluten intolerance and celiac disease. Those conditions include type 1 diabetes, autoimmune thyroid diseases, Hashimoto's disease, Graves' disease, and Addison's disease.

Any person, child or adult, with gluten intolerance and celiac disease should be screened for osteoporosis and the presence of autoimmune diseases. The risk of occurrence of these conditions is increased when you have an associated or predisposing disorder. An additional diagnostic problem is the wide variety of symptoms related to gluten intolerance and celiac disease. A person with gluten intolerance and celiac disease may not show the classical symptoms of abdominal pain, diarrhea, constipation, and malabsorption. The only sign of underlying celiac disease may be infertility or hyperthyroidism.

These possibilities make diagnosis difficult for physicians who are less than familiar with gluten intolerance and celiac disease. Physicians and the public need an increased awareness of these conditions. In particular, physicians need to become more conversant with the features of gluten intolerance and celiac disease and they need to raise the level of their diagnostic capabilities. Additionally, they need to learn how to look beyond the features of day-to-day cases and consider unusual circumstances and less-common conditions.

The Cancer Connection

Hearing the News

"I remember everything about that day," said Gary Cartwright describing the day his doctor told him he had cancer. "I'd already had a lot of health issues. Eventually you think you just can't take any more." Gary sat a little straighter in his chair and looked directly at his questioner. "But what can you do? You have to go on."

Gary Cartwright, 52 years old, is a real estate executive with more than 25 years experience in San Diego County. "I majored in English literature at UCLA. Met a girl. Got married. Things don't always work out like you planned." He smiled. "Two sets of twins two years apart," he added. "Having four kids after only four years of marriage will concentrate your mind in a hurry."

Gary had a loving family and was building his reputation and getting known up and down Highways 5 and 15 in Southern California, but in his early thirties things started to go wrong with his health. "The joints in my hands became swollen and painful, then the pain spread to my wrists and I thought I was going to become disabled." He had difficulty holding a cup of coffee and opening a jar of salsa or tomato sauce was excruciating. "Uncorking a bottle of wine?" he asked rhetorically. "Forget it."

Gary thought he had some unusual form of early arthritis. "Arthritis runs in my family, but what do I know? What I do know is that I don't like going to doctors." He refused to see his family doctor and when the pain worsened he increased his dosage of over-the-counter pain pills. "Then the fevers started and I began to think I had a real problem."

"I was running hot and cold and Clare, my wife, would joke that I was having hot flashes. At the time I didn't think she was being very funny." In addition, Gary had developed blotches on his face. "Sounds to me like lupus," said a friend who was a resident in internal medicine at UCSD School of Medicine. "You'd better see your doctor." Gary called his doctor that day. "I didn't want to go because I knew that first visit wouldn't be the last, not by a long shot, but I went anyway."

Gary's doctor confirmed the suspicion of lupus and drew blood for a battery of tests which were reasonably conclusive. Gary's blood contained antinuclear antibodies (ANA) and his sedimentation rate (ESR) was elevated, indicating an active inflammatory process. ANA are also found in other autoimmune diseases including rheumatoid arthritis, autoimmune hepatitis, and scleroderma.

"My doctor said I was anemic and asked if I'd been feeling tired or worn-out," Gary added. "I told him I'd been too worried to really notice, but yeah, if I had to think about it, I was pretty knocked out." His doctor told him anemia is another sign of lupus and the combination of joint pains, fever, anemia, and facial rash suggested lupus as the main problem.

"They started me on steroids to control the symptoms and help me get stronger. The drugs weren't much fun, but I did start to feel better. They put me on a low-fat diet and told me to stay out of the sun." Gary's doctors had a good management plan. Plaquenil, an antiparasitic and immunosuppressant commonly prescribed to treat lupus was introduced to control symptoms. He tolerated it well and was encouraged to do mild to moderate exercise. Gary survived past the ten-year mark, which was a good thing for someone with lupus.

Gary never mentioned his bouts of diarrhea and abdominal pain and none of his doctors thought to ask about gastrointestinal complaints. They were doing a good job, focusing on the typical rheumatological symptoms of lupus and attempting to prevent cardiovascular and kidney problems as well as other consequences, but no one considered the possibility of additional, seemingly unrelated disorders that might have contributed to the development of lupus in the first place.

Gary had lived with gastrointestinal issues since he was a teenager and for him, periodic abdominal pain and diarrhea were in the category of "stuff happens." His symptoms came and went. They were briefly unpleasant, then they were gone. Most teenagers don't obsess about their health and Gary was typical. He always had a lot going on and once college started he became even busier. Even as a young adult he never connected the dots and never recognized that his abdominal symptoms always happened after random pizza parties or family events where he ate cake and cookies, things he usually didn't eat.

Over time Gary's gastrointestinal complaints became worse. He had more frequent abdominal pains and the pain was increasing. Diarrhea became more frequent and he had abdominal bloating. Clare suggested he keep a diary and Gary started documenting what he ate every day along with his daily activities and the presence of any abdominal symptoms. Eventually Clare and Gary observed a pattern. Whenever he ate bread, pizza, or pasta he had problems. Cookies, cake, and pie also gave him trouble.

"I never liked bread that much when I was a kid," Gary said. "Pizza, that was in the same category, and for some reason I wasn't a cake-and-cookies fan. I guess I was weird. Chocolate? Now that I liked. Ice cream, too. Any flavor. I just wasn't a bread man."

Do-It-Yourself Research

Gary and Clare did some research and found out about gluten intolerance and celiac disease. The symptoms caused by gluten intolerance were similar to Gary's gastrointestinal complaints. As they continued learning about celiac disease, they discovered that it could be associated with other diseases, including lupus. Gary remembered his teenage episodes of diarrhea and abdominal pain and questioned whether those things might have been the start of his future health problems. He wondered if his lupus might have been slowed or even avoided altogether with proper attention back then, but Clare reminded him that hindsight is always 20/20. The important thing was to get his current problems fixed and become as healthy as possible.

Gary made an appointment to see his rheumatologist, but his doctor didn't give much credence to Gary's ideas. "One thing doesn't have anything to do with the other," the doctor told him. "Don't believe everything you read on the Internet." Gary left the office with a referral to a gastroenterologist who also took a dim view of Gary's research. "Leave medicine to the specialists," was this doctor's sage advice. He ordered a barium study of the upper gastrointestinal tract and prescribed Imodium for the diarrhea. Gary didn't follow through on either of these recommendations and his abdominal symptoms persisted.

Clare believed they could find a knowledgeable physician and launched a phone and email campaign. Within a week they had a recommendation to see a new rheumatologist. "I thought we were looking for a gastroenterologist," Gary said to Clare. "That's what I thought, too," she replied, "but apparently we need to see a specialist in autoimmune diseases."

At the first appointment we asked Gary in-depth disease-oriented questions, and he immediately felt he was in the right place. "I felt the doctor was engaging me rather than talking at me," Gary said. "He seemed to want to know about *me*, not only about my symptoms." A few days later the lab tests came back positive for specific autoimmune findings. Next, Gary went for a biopsy of his small intestine, which showed the characteristic changes of celiac disease.

We gave Gary the news and told him about the need for a strict gluten-free diet. "It was actually a relief," he recalled. "At least now all the cards were on the table." He learned about the relationship between celiac disease and additional autoimmune disorders.

After a few months of his new gluten-free diet, Gary's abdominal symptoms had largely resolved. He no longer experienced abdominal pain and diarrhea had become an unusual occurrence. "A big bonus was that I was having fewer lupus flares. My hands felt better and I was able to reduce the dosage of all my medications. I felt a lot stronger being on the gluten-free diet, but then the other shoe dropped."

We had emphasized to Gary the need for consistent follow-up. It was important to be watchful for the development of other conditions, particularly certain malignancies of the gastrointestinal tract. "I had read about this during all the research Clare and I had done," Gary said. "Still, it's easy to forget about stuff like that. You think it's not going to happen to you."

Following our advice, Gary went for periodic re-examinations during the next few years. These follow-ups consisted of blood tests and physical exams, and as Gary said, "They weren't that big a deal, until he began to experiencing a recurrence of abdominal pain and fatigue. His next follow-up exam was a month away, but Gary called to see if he could come in early which was a good idea because the new examination showed something different.

"I was anemic and some other blood tests were positive," Gary said. "Dr. Shikhman told me that any return of symptoms is suspicious if you've been on a gluten-free diet for a long time." He was referred to an oncologist and underwent a biopsy, CT scan, and additional blood tests. "Bottom line—they told me I had non-Hodgkin's lymphoma. That was very tough to hear."

"Even so, there was good news," Gary continued. "Thankfully I'd been going for all the follow-ups, and they caught the cancer early. Otherwise I don't know where I'd be. I did radiation and chemo. Now we're waiting, but I've gone back to work and I'm feeling pretty good again. One more thing," he added. "I don't know what my future holds, but I do know this: being told to go on a gluten-free diet was the best medical advice I ever got."

Gluten Intolerance, Celiac Disease, and the Risk of Malignancy

> **Non-Hodgkin's lymphoma** (NHL) is a hematologic cancer derived from lymphocytes — white blood cells. There are many types of NHL characterized by the type of lymphocyte involved. Both B-cell lymphoma and T-cell lymphoma can be found in patients with celiac disease.

People with gluten intolerance and celiac disease have an increased risk of developing certain malignancies. Their overall risk of cancer is almost twice that of the general population. These cancers include non-Hodgkin's lymphoma, carcinoma of the small intestine, pharyngeal (throat) carcinoma, cancers of the liver and pancreas, and melanoma. The causes of these associations are not known with certainty, but the relationships have been proven over many decades.

Cancers are composed of cells whose growth and reproduction don't respond to normal regulatory and feedback systems. In other words, the growth and reproduction of cancer cells are no longer under the control of the host. Normally these processes are tightly regulated, but cancer doesn't respond to the host's signaling mechanisms. Cancer cells are smart, creative, highly adaptive, and expand locally, displacing the surrounding normal tissue. There's no unused space in the body, so the displaced normal tissue atrophies with a resulting loss of function. Additionally, the pressure exerted by the cancer on normal tissue causes pain which can be constant and intense, often worsening at night owing to the absence of distractions present during the day. Once a cancer reaches a certain size, the pain produced by pressure on surrounding tissues can be unrelenting.

Malignant cancers can grow their own blood supply, a process known as angiogenesis which facilitates a tumor's growth by increasing nutrient availability. Spread of the tumor to other parts of the body, known as metastasis, is enabled via transmission of tumor cells through the new system of blood vessels. Malignant cancers cause a variety of health problems in addition to local pain and loss of function of surrounding tissues. The life of a cancer is literally stolen from the host itself by hijacking supplies of oxygen and other nutrients designated for delivery to normal host tissues. These diverted nutrients feed the cancer instead of the host, and if the cancer is large enough the host's health suffers. Characteristic signs of malignancy such as unexpected weight loss are due to this ongoing diversion of nutrients to a growing cancer. Chronic fatigue is another sign, owing to lack of nutrition as well as the person's ongoing battle against pain.

Cancers are named and categorized based on the type of tissue from which they arise. A **carcinoma** is a malignant cancer of *epithelium*. Epithelial cells line the cavities of hollow organs such as the stomach and intestines, cover the surface of structures such as the skin, and form glands such as the thyroid gland and pancreas.

Understanding of the *process* of cancer — why cancers appear and how they grow and develop has been changing in recent years. In the past, cancers were considered entities such as breast cancer, lung cancer, and colon cancer. Although these are all carcinomas, they were considered different. One person might have bone cancer, an example of a *sarcoma* (a malignancy of connective tissue such as bone, cartilage, and muscle). Another might have a *rhabdomyosarcoma*, a rare malignancy of muscle seen in childhood.

These tumors all have distinct appearances under the microscope. For the most part they can be easily distinguished by any medical student, but they're all cancers and their shared characteristics are more important than their differences. Modern cancer specialists acknowledge that cancers as a group represent a continuum of disorders. The particular cancer affecting an individual occupies a place at a certain point in time, demonstrating more of certain characteristics versus others, but what's most important is that the disorder is a cancer that represents a breakdown in the functioning of that individual.

Most malignancies are difficult to treat and a malignant tumor may never truly die. Traditional treatment of a malignancy involves radiation, chemotherapy, and surgery. Radiation is employed to kill the cancer cells and is highly effective, but it's never certain whether all the tumor cells are destroyed. Surgery removes a large section of tissue that contains the tumor, but certain types of tumor may have metastasized, spreading undetectable seeds that may later develop into clinically significant lesions. Chemotherapy kills cells that reproduce rapidly like malignant cancer cells, but chemotherapy is not specific and kills all cells that have a rapid turnover rate, such as white blood cells, cells lining the gastrointestinal tract, and hair follicle cells.

These blunt instruments have been the only armaments available in the war against cancer, and the more we learn, the more complex the overall problem seems to be. Cancer researchers now know that classifications such as *breast cancer* or *colon cancer* are far too simplistic. A block of tissue from a malignant tumor of the breast may contain thousands of genetic variants. The cells are *not alike* and the genetic structure of malignant cells is *highly unstable*. Owing to their rapid rate of reproduction, mutations are common. A drug that kills some tumor cells will not kill all of them, as some cells are genetically resistant. The resistant cells will multiply and the tumor will become more resistant. Attempts to kill cancers literally become an arms race.

Recent findings are encouraging. Research in the relatively new field of lifestyle medicine shows that a significant proportion of cancers are in fact lifestyle disorders. Approximately 40% of all cancers are caused by deleterious lifestyle choices. The implication is that frequently, cancer is a preventable disease.

Causes of Cancer Associated with Gluten Intolerance and Celiac Disease

Scientists have searched for the causes of cancer for decades. It is now generally recognized that the causes of cancer arise from a combination of factors. Genetic, environmental, and even socioeconomic factors act together to cause cancer in person A. Person B, the coworker or neighbor does not develop cancer as a different set of factors are in play.

Exposure to high levels of radiation causes cancer, but not everyone in the exposed group develops it. Those who do not may have inherited certain genetic patterns that lend protection. Alternatively, they may gain protection from lifelong habits of a healthful diet and exercise. Similarly, not every construction worker exposed to asbestos develops *mesothelioma* (a carcinoma most commonly found in the *pleura*, the outer lining of the lungs).

Internal and external environmental causes may play a role in the development of cancer in gluten intolerance and celiac disease. The main environmental factor is exposure to gluten itself. In genetically susceptible individuals, ingestion of gluten provokes a cascade of immunologic responses. Over time, with prolonged exposure to gluten, the immunologic responses in turn cause an extensive inflammatory reaction. It is well known that chronic inflammation can lead to malignant transformation of previously normal cells and tissues.

Chronic inflammation of the gallbladder can lead to gallbladder carcinoma. Chronic and repeated bladder infections with accompanying inflammation can lead to cancer of the bladder. Chronic inflammation of the liver (possibly due to alcohol, drug overuse, or abuse) can cause hepatic carcinoma (cancer of the liver). Chronic inflammation of the stomach (possibly a result of stomach ulcers) can cause gastric carcinoma (stomach cancer). Specific malignant transformation of chronic inflammation of the small intestine (such as in gluten intolerance and celiac disease) can occur, but is uncommon.

In gluten intolerance and celiac disease, additional cancers can develop in the small intestine and other locations in the gastrointestinal tract. Non-Hodgkin's lymphoma and carcinoma of the stomach, throat, or mouth are examples of such malignant tumors. Chronic immunological stimulation and reaction, resulting from chronic ingestion of gluten is a likely cause of these lesions. There are numerous explanations, including development of an autoimmune response. In the case of carcinomas, the immune system attacks tissues of the gastrointestinal tract, which encounters gluten on a chronic basis and subclinical inflammation develops. There are no overt symptoms, but a low-grade inflammatory reaction results, ultimately causing a malignant change in the affected tissue. Non-Hodgkin's lymphoma probably results from chronic immunological stimulation. T cells and B cells are both significant participants in the immunological cascade provoked by consumption of gluten-containing foods. T cell and B cell clones are created in the small intestine producing identical cells that respond to a specific immunological stimulus. Some cell lines can mutate and develop the ability to ignore regulatory signals and reproduce at will. These cell lines become lymphomas.

> **T cells** are lymphocytes — white blood cells — that have an array of immunological functions. Helper T cells assist other immunological cells such as B cells. Once a helper T cell has recognized a foreign protein, the helper T cell activates a specific B cell. Regulatory T cells help shut down an immune response once it has served its purpose.
>
> **B cells** are lymphocytes that produce antibodies to a specific foreign protein after they have been activated by a specific T cell.

Increased Risk of Cancer in Gluten Intolerance and Celiac Disease

Many studies have demonstrated the increased risk of cancer in people with gluten intolerance and celiac disease. Reports were first published more than 50 years ago. Studies from this period suggested a 100-fold increased risk of non-Hodgkin's lymphoma in patients with celiac disease. Although the risk for non-Hodgkin's lymphoma is significant, the estimation of risk has been decreasing owing to a variety of factors. At present, a nine-fold increased risk represents a reasonable assessment.

A famous, frequently cited study was published in the peer-reviewed journal Gut in 1989 that described a group of 210 patients with celiac disease who had been followed for more than 11 years. The results indicate that for celiac patients on a gluten-free diet for five years or more, the risk of developing cancer is not increased compared to the general population, but the risk is increased in those taking a reduced gluten or a normal diet. Thirty-eight patients developed a malignant cancer during the study period, representing a doubling of the overall risk of the general population. Nine patients had non-Hodgkin's lymphoma, representing a 43-fold increased incidence. Three had cancer of the esophagus, representing a 12-fold increase. Three patients had cancer of the mouth and throat, representing a 10-fold increase compared with the general population. This well-known study found that a gluten-free diet offered protection against malignancy in patients with gluten intolerance and celiac disease. The authors recommended that all such patients go on a gluten-free diet for life.

With respect to lymphoma, a study conducted in Scotland was reported in 1989. Investigation of 653 patients with celiac disease revealed a 30-fold increase in risk of developing a lymphoma-type disease. A study done in Italy reported on 1000 patients with celiac disease referred by specialist clinics. In this group, non-Hodgkin's lymphoma was found at a rate almost 70 times greater than expected. In contrast, another study done in Italy reported in 2002 investigated 653 patients with lymphoma. The authors identified a risk of 3.1 of developing non-Hodgkin's lymphoma in patients with celiac disease.

The present estimate of a two-fold overall risk of developing cancer in patients with gluten intolerance and celiac disease compared to that of the general population remains a substantial risk. There have been numerous reports of higher risk levels. In the case of lymphoma, reported risks have varied widely, and as we've seen, these differences can be attributed to several factors.

Studies done from the 1960s through the early 1990s involved small groups of patients evaluated in specialty clinics who were a subset of all those with celiac disease. These patients were sufficiently ill to require treatment in hospitals. Publications describing a many-fold increase in risk for cancer were based on the presence of cancer in those patients with celiac disease who were already sick. The data became skewed not only owing to the small numbers of patients involved, but also because these patients were not representative of the entire group of people with gluten intolerance and celiac disease. Technically, these earlier data sets have limited statistical power. More statistically, valid investigations were needed involving larger groups of people. Such studies are known as population studies that evaluate a group of patients (a *cohort*) that demonstrate the full range of symptoms of celiac disease. Some cases are mild, others more severe. This is a key statistical benefit. Small studies tend to include only those at one end of the spectrum and the results are less applicable overall.

A **standardized incidence ratio** (SIR) is the ratio of the observed number of cases in a study compared to the expected number based on the risk in the general population. For example, a certain disease occurs with a frequency of $1/1,000$ in the general population. In a study of 1,000 subjects, four persons have the disease. The SIR is 4.0 (4:1).

In an attempt to develop data with greater predictive power, researchers in Sweden followed 11,000 persons with celiac disease. The average follow-up period was approximately ten years. The study was published in 2002 and reported a *standardized incidence ratio* (SIR) of cancer equal to 1.3. This risk level is many times lower than those reported in smaller studies and even lower than the two-fold overall increase in cancer risk for patients with celiac disease currently in use.

Important differences in risk were identified. The SIR for developing lymphoma in those first hospitalized with celiac disease during childhood (younger than age 10) was 1.4, but for those first hospitalized with celiac disease when they were older than age 20, the SIR for developing lymphoma was considerably higher: 7.0. This level of lymphoma risk appears appropriate and statistically valid.

Ascertainment bias is another consideration relating to historically elevated risk levels for development of malignancy in celiac disease. In ascertainment bias, the eligible population is not defined appropriately. In earlier studies the onset of lymphoma can in some cases, cause symptoms of celiac disease in persons in whom celiac disease had been previously silent. In other words, lymphoma provoked the development of celiac disease symptoms. These silent cases are added to the known cases of celiac disease with lymphoma that lead to an overestimation of the overall risk.

The converse of this is known as *detection bias* in which a person with undetected celiac disease manifests symptoms and becomes a known case of celiac disease, but these symptoms developed owing to an underlying, not-yet-diagnosed malignancy. In a short period of time, the lymphoma or other malignancy is also diagnosed, skewing the calculation of the risk factor for the particular cancer in celiac disease. Any of these factors can lead to overestimation of the risk of developing malignancy in persons with celiac disease.

A contemporary source of the reduction in risk is attributed to recent advancements in the diagnosis of celiac disease. Earlier diagnosis is possible owing to improved laboratory testing (identification of immunological markers in patients' blood samples), as well as earlier adoption of and greater adherence to a gluten-free diet which reduces a person's exposure to gluten. Healing begins soon after starting a gluten-free diet and continues as long as the patient remains gluten free.

The risk for developing malignancy increases the longer celiac disease remains undiagnosed. In those with undetected and untreated gluten intolerance and celiac disease, immunological responses and inflammatory reactions continue unchecked. A study done in Italy reported in 2007 followed 1,968 patients with celiac disease. The average age of diagnosis of celiac disease for patients who developed intestinal non-Hodgkin's lymphoma was 47.6. The average age of diagnosis for those who did not was 28.6. Earlier adoption of effective treatment puts the brakes on immunological responses and inflammatory reactions, reducing an important risk factor.

Increasing awareness of the clinical characteristics of gluten intolerance and celiac disease, particularly among primary care physicians, will lead to greater detection and timely treatment. As many cases of celiac disease show atypical signs and symptoms and can have no associated abdominal and gastrointestinal symptoms, an increased index of suspicion among physicians of all specialties is needed for accurate diagnosis and intervention.

When to Suspect a Possible Malignancy

In general, the presence of cancer is associated with a significant change in normal patterns of health. Weight loss for no apparent reason, a sudden and persistent alteration in bowel habits, an unexplained and persistent loss of appetite, pronounced fatigue, and alterations in sleep habits are all suggestive of the development of a malignant disorder. The presence of one or several of these symptoms doesn't suggest that a person *has* cancer, but that a diagnosis of malignancy should be carefully evaluated.

Patients with celiac disease who are on a gluten-free diet usually experience symptomatic improvement or resolution. Unexplained deterioration in such patients should alert the treating physician to the possibility of malignancy. The development of weight loss, fever, muscular fatigue, and swollen lymph nodes should strongly suggest the presence of lymphoma. If the patient's deterioration also includes malaise, diarrhea, and abdominal pain, the specific type of lymphoma may be enteropathy-associated T-cell lymphoma. The development of new symptoms and/or the recurrence of abdominal pain and diarrhea in a patient on a gluten-free diet should always necessitate a thorough reevaluation.

Protective Benefits of a Gluten-Free Diet with Respect to Malignancy

Early studies from the late 1980s showed there was *no significant increase* in overall cancer risk for patients with celiac disease who were on a strict gluten-free diet for more than five years. For those patients with celiac disease who were not on a strict gluten-free diet, there was a *significantly increased risk* of malignancy.

A mid-1990s study conducted in Finland reported no cases of non-Hodgkin's lymphoma in a group of 335 celiac patients who were diagnosed early, 83% of whom were compliant with a gluten-free diet. A report published in 2003 suggested that much of the cancer risk associated with celiac disease occurs before the condition is diagnosed. The risk going forward is reduced by the patient's beginning and staying on a gluten-free diet. The authors indicate that earlier diagnosis and a strict gluten-free diet will likely reduce the risk of malignancy in celiac disease. A study published in 2008 suggested that a strict gluten-free diet provides protection against the development of gastrointestinal lymphoma.

Some researchers advocate an even more proactive approach. Research published in 1997 studied 8,690 secondary school students in Italy. The authors of the study recommended a gluten-free diet for individuals with silent celiac disease—those persons with positive laboratory tests but no symptoms. The authors stated that even apparently silent celiac disease is not truly "silent." After starting a gluten-free diet, young people in this study reported height and weight gains, improvement in appetite and mood, improved physical fitness, and improved performance in school. These significant enhancements in physical health and quality of life affirm the importance of a gluten-free diet in all cases of celiac disease, silent or otherwise. Treatment of asymptomatic celiac disease with a gluten-free diet may help prevent long-term complications of celiac disease including: anemia, infertility, malignancy, and osteoporosis.

For individuals with gluten intolerance and celiac disease, a gluten-free diet for life is likely to provide protective benefits with respect to malignancy and many other chronic diseases. Greater awareness among physicians and the public, earlier diagnosis of celiac disease, and greater adherence to a gluten-free diet will significantly improve the long-term health of all individuals with gluten intolerance and celiac disease.

The Science of Gluten Intolerance and Celiac Disease

Out of Darkness

Tracy Monroe was running out of time. At age 52, every day seemed more troublesome than the day before. Tracy had suffered health issues for many years and felt as if her little store of energy was slipping away. Even the pleasure she gained from her children was poor compensation for putting up with her increasing pain and discomfort. Thoughts of suicide were gaining strength and mechanical talismans like shaking her head or blinking her eyes had lost their effectiveness in dispelling her darkness. Tracy stood at the edge of an abyss and was losing the will to keep herself from falling in until one morning when she read an article in the *San Diego Union-Tribune* that seemed to have been written expressly for her.

Rheumatoid arthritis had been her main tormentor. She had received this diagnosis 15 years earlier when she was 37 years old when her daughter was 15 and her son was 3. With a teenager and a young child at home, her day was filled with responsibilities. There was no room in Tracy's life for health problems.

When recalling her childhood, she described herself as a sickly kid who always had a lot of colds, was never really healthy, and had constant pains in her stomach as well as frequent episodes of bloating and diarrhea.

"When you grow up not feeling good you don't know how bad you really feel," she said. "You don't know you don't feel good. I wasn't as sharp mentally as the other kids." She would wake up groggy and feel as if she never got enough sleep. She didn't have as much energy as her friends and tired easily. Concerning her menstrual cycle, Tracy said, "My period was real heavy and I could never track it on a calendar like other girls." She described an unusual 14 days of flow during some cycles and 6 days of flow during others. Her menstrual cycle never became consistent and she never knew what to expect.

She became pregnant for the first time when she was 22 and by the beginning of her second trimester, Tracy experienced increasing stomach pain and abdominal bloating. She was either constipated or had diarrhea and her obstetrician referred her for a colonoscopy. Tracy did some reading on her own and thought she might have celiac disease, but her doctor informed her "there is no celiac disease in America," and diagnosed irritable bowel syndrome. Tracy's symptoms continued until a friend recommended consulting a nutritionist. When Tracy began a more balanced diet based on the nutritionist's recommendations, her abdominal symptoms improved.

Symptoms of rheumatoid arthritis began during her second pregnancy, but because this pregnancy was so difficult, her joint problems were overlooked. "I never really felt healthy before I became pregnant," she said, but felt even worse once pregnant. "I took a turn for the worse right away," she said, describing constant diarrhea and stomach pains, sometimes accompanied by fever. She had difficulty sleeping and became agitated. "My health was going down the tubes and I couldn't stop it."

During the early stage of this pregnancy her thumbs began to feel sore, and this pain was soon followed by pain in her fingers, wrists, elbows, and lower back. "I thought I was going crazy." She remembered undergoing a complete personality change, becoming depressed and considering suicide many times, but her baby came first.

Tracy's joint pain subsided after her delivery, but returned a few years later. Rheumatoid arthritis was diagnosed. Her doctors prescribed Remicade, an immunosuppressant, Plaquenil, and methotrexate injections, another immunosuppressant used in chemotherapy. Tracy never felt well with Remicade. "I was constantly fighting the side effects of whatever medication I was on." Her joints remained swollen and painful. In addition, she suffered other health issues including, really bad periods, severe anemia, low adrenals, a low thyroid, and several bouts of pneumonia.

After nine or ten years of various treatments and therapies, Tracy's own medical opinion was that "an underlying problem was being overlooked. Her investigations and readings suggested celiac disease as a major cause, but her doctors refused to consider the possibility. One physician told her that celiac disease doesn't exist. Another stated there was "no way" that celiac disease was the problem. She decided to go off all her arthritis medications and experienced more joint pain, then she lost mobility and her fevers returned. She felt she was reaching the end of the road when she read an article in the *Healthy Times* written by Dr. Shikhman describing the symptoms and treatment of celiac disease. Tracy felt both relief and hope for the first time in years and scheduled an appointment for the required tests which resulted in a diagnosis of celiac disease. Tracy began to believe she was finally in the right place.

She immediately started a gluten free diet and her abdominal symptoms, including pain, diarrhea, constipation, and bloating, began to clear up right away. Tracy had been experiencing "brain fog" for several years prior to beginning the gluten-free diet and was very forthcoming about her long periods of depression and her thoughts of suicide.

"I track all these mental problems back to my second pregnancy, when my stomach symptoms got much worse and the joint pains began. As soon as I started the gluten-free diet my mind became a lot sharper. I could think straight for the first time in a long time. I'm not depressed any more. That's all behind me. In fact, I have a pretty normal quality of life right now thanks to Dr. Shikhman and my gluten-free diet."

We also made several other recommendations designed to get Tracy feeling better right away. We started her on Prednisone to get the worst of the rheumatoid arthritis symptoms under control. She said the treatment with Prednisone was great. We also prescribed Plaquenil, but it had unacceptable side effects including hair loss. Tracy discontinued it and her rheumatoid arthritis symptoms worsened. Something else was needed, so we started her on Rituxan (Rituximab), a type of antibody drug and biological agent that is given intravenously which stopped all symptoms, including fever, joint pain, joint swelling, and other symptoms of rheumatoid arthritis.

Tracy said that her first Christmas after starting our treatment program was the best holiday season she'd experienced in a very long time. "I felt present and could actually enjoy things." She continued on Prednisone for five months. Her Rituxan protocol was to receive two intravenous treatments separated by two weeks, then wait six months before the next round which worked very well. She felt pretty normal, had no side effects, and her hair grew back. She has no more symptoms of rheumatoid arthritis. She had gone through 12 long, discouraging, and debilitating years before finally finding an effective treatment.

A visitor at our clinic asked Tracy about tips for going on a gluten-free diet. "My tastes have changed quite a bit since I started my diet," she said. "I have so many choices. I can have everything everyone else is eating. All I need to do is make sure my dishes are gluten-free."

"The information about going on a gluten-free diet was empowering," she continued. "I look at what I *can* eat. I focus on the positive. For me gluten means *pain*, so it was an easy transition. I'm striving to get better so I want to avoid anything that contains gluten. It's so nice to be able to eat and not have anything wrong with me afterward. Once you get past your mental barriers, you learn where it's safe to eat out. The way I look at it, I feel fortunate and happy if there's something on the menu I can eat."

When the visitor said that being on a gluten-free diet sounded pretty easy, Tracy said, "Well, there's definitely a learning curve. When your doctor says you have celiac disease and need to go on a gluten-free diet, that's a lot to take in all at once, besides you're physically sick, mentally worn out, and overwhelmed by everything that's been happening to you. In the beginning, I was scared there wouldn't be anything that I could eat. I lost weight and got really thin, down to 110 pounds, then I finally got it together and now I have a normal outlook. I know what I'm doing. I call manufacturers if I'm not sure about a certain product. I call ahead to restaurants if we're going out for breakfast or dinner. Being on a gluten-free diet is really simple. It's a very healthy way to eat."

Tracy emphasized the full extent of her recovery. "I'm in complete remission thanks to Dr. Shikhman's expert care. I have some permanent deformities due to the rheumatoid arthritis, but now I can actually use my hands. Doctors need to think about the cause, the root, of a person's problems. People don't understand why doctors only look at the symptoms. I saw so many doctors, but I never found a doctor like Dr. Shikhman who covers the whole thing for you. He's the only real doctor I've ever had in my life."

Tracy's medical history demonstrates a strong relationship between gluten intolerance, celiac disease, and rheumatoid arthritis. Her history also shows a strong link between gluten intolerance, celiac disease, and neuropsychiatric disorders like clinical depression and suicidal ideation. Gluten intolerance and celiac disease may also have impacted Tracy's family. Her daughter is unable to have children owing to a congenital abnormality. Her son has ADHD and problems with his vision. As we've seen, celiac disease can cause problems for the mother during pregnancy, and these may lead to health problems for the children of those pregnancies.

A Look Under the Hood

We will now take an in-depth look at the science behind gluten intolerance and celiac disease which has caused of so much suffering for people like Tracy. During the last 50 years celiac disease has become recognized as a common condition affecting approximately one in 100 persons. The large majority of these people remain undiagnosed. Raising public awareness and improving the medical profession's understanding of gluten intolerance and celiac disease are two major health priorities.

Receiving an accurate diagnosis and beginning appropriate treatment without delay are important considerations when a person seeks medical advice. An additional concern is the possibility of long-term complications of undiagnosed and untreated gluten intolerance and celiac disease. Awareness and understanding are important, particularly as gluten intolerance and celiac disease are such great mimickers of other disorders and may not present with classical, easily recognizable signs and symptoms.

Gluten intolerance and celiac disease represent a continuum of physiological responses to gluten that begins with an immunological reaction. As the gluten-intolerant person's exposure continues, the immunological response progresses and can spread to other systems in addition to the gastrointestinal tract where the immunological response provokes an inflammatory reaction. When actual damage is done to the lining of the small intestine, the disorder can be termed celiac disease.

Many pieces of the puzzle remain misunderstood, yet robust models can successfully account for the facts. The effective treatment of a gluten-free diet for life has been known for many years. The scientific background is now filling in and helping to explain why a gluten-free diet works and why it needs to be implemented as quickly as possible.

Gluten, Wheat, and Celiac Disease

Gluten proteins comprise approximately 80% of the protein contained in wheat and provides nourishment to the developing plant. It may also help protect the seedlings against drought. Gluten also makes wheat an excellent cereal for baking. Gluten proteins provide desirable consistency and elasticity to dough, making the finished product palatable and delicious. There are 10,000 known varieties of wheat and a single wheat variety can contain 100 different gluten proteins. Gluten is also found in other dietary grains including barley and rye.

Many recent studies have shown that in a genetically susceptible individual, duration of exposure to gluten is strongly correlated with development of additional diseases such as malignancy and autoimmune disorders. Studies in young children have demonstrated that exposure to gluten before the age of 6 months is related to development of gluten intolerance and celiac disease. Two important conclusions can be drawn from these findings.

1. Wheat, barley, and rye containing foods should not be given to infants younger than 6 months of age. After 6 months, they can slowly introduced to these foods. These recommendations contrast with the typical diet of most babies who are given unrestricted access to gluten-containing foods, a circumstance that often initiates the process of gluten intolerance.

2. Early diagnosis of gluten intolerance and celiac disease restores quality of life and helps prevent long-term complications.

How Does Gluten Provoke an Immunological Response?

Basic Structure of the Gastrointestinal (GI) Tract

The GI tract is a hollow tube. The space within the tube is the *lumen*. The wall of the tube surrounding the lumen is a three-layered structure of varying thickness. The outer layer — the *serosa* — is the protective covering. The middle layer contains contractile involuntary muscle that pushes food down the tract. The inner layer — the *mucosa* — contains the *epithelium* and the *lamina propria*. The epithelium is a specialized layer of cells that do the work of digestion. The lamina propria is a layer of supporting cells and tissues. In the small intestine the lamina propria contains capillaries, lymphatic vessels, and lymphoid tissue that produces lymphocytes (specialized white blood cells).

We need to consume protein to remain healthy and well. Gluten is a complex of proteins that are key components of whole grains, a major food group. Our gastrointestinal tracts are designed to digest proteins. Why does gluten cause so many problems for so many people?

Composed of proteins that are not completely digestible by humans, rather than getting broken down into individual amino acids in the gastrointestinal tract, gluten is only partially digested into large fragments which can:

- Be excreted and cause no problems.
- Persist in the small intestine, interacting with the epithelial cells and provoking an *innate* immunological response in susceptible individuals.
- Penetrate the lamina propria and provoke an *adaptive* immunological response in susceptible individuals.

In genetically susceptible individuals, gluten provokes both an innate and an adaptive immunological response.

Innate Immunity and Adaptive Immunity

Humans possess both an inborn immunity to a range of microorganisms and foreign proteins and an adaptive immunity that can produce an on-the-fly immunological response to foreign proteins and microorganisms. Innate immunity is a built-in system. Adaptive immunity is acquired, similar to on-the-job experience.

Innate immunity is similar to an army's first-line of defense. Many microorganisms are prevented from invading human tissues by the *epithelium*, the cells lining the gastrointestinal tract and other mucous membranes. These structural epithelial barriers are part of innate immunity. *Natural killer cells* and *macrophages* are also components of innate immunity. Natural killer cells are specialized lymphocytes and macrophages are specialized white blood cells. These cells work together to attack and kill microorganisms that have breached the epithelial defenses. Natural killer cells also kill virus-infected host cells.

Adaptive immunity is a slower-acting system with greater flexibility and range of responses that can adapt to enable its forces to combat new, never-before-experienced pathogens. Many microorganisms have developed the ability to evade destruction by the processes of innate immunity. The adaptive immune system has the capability of learning how to destroy these "smart" pathogens.

The adaptive immune system consists of T lymphocytes and B lymphocytes. T lymphocytes mature in the *thymus*, an organ located in the center of the chest behind the sternum. B lymphocytes mature in the bone marrow. T lymphocytes are subdivided into helper T cells and cytotoxic (cell-killing) T cells. CD4+ helper T cells help B lymphocytes produce antibodies and help macrophages kill microorganisms. A specialized subset of CD4+ helper T cells limit and shutdown the immune response. These are regulatory T cells. CD8+ T cells are cytotoxic T cells that kill infected host cells.

Foreign proteins contained in the cells of a transplanted kidney or heart are also antigens. For an organ transplant to be successful, the immune response of the host must be weakened with immunosuppressive drugs. Normally the host's B lymphocytes would produce many antibodies against the transplanted organ's proteins. Immunosuppressive drugs help to minimize this response and allow the transplanted tissue to become incorporated successfully into the host.

B lymphocytes manufacture antibodies that recognize specific foreign proteins. A foreign protein is an *antigen* which can be found on the surface of invading microorganisms. Other antigens are metabolic products of the invaders. *Antibodies* produced by B lymphocytes have specialized regions designed to bind specific antigens. The binding site is highly variable and millions of antibodies can be produced, each of which will bind to a specific foreign protein. By binding to an antigen on a foreign cell's surface, the antibody marks that cell for destruction. Antibodies can also bind to foreign proteins circulating in the blood. These antigen-antibody complexes are engulfed by phagocytes, yet another type of specialized white blood cell that engulfs and absorbs bacteria and other small cells and particles.

Innate immunity is a rapid-response system designed to combat infections. It can slow the effects of virulent pathogens until adaptive immunity is activated. There is extensive cross-talk between these two systems. Each provides information to the other to help facilitate immune responses, increase efficiency of response, and protect the host.

Friendly Fire: The Development of Autoimmune Diseases

The function of innate immunity and adaptive immunity is to protect the host against invading microorganisms, toxic foreign pathogens, and tumor cells. The immune system does this by distinguishing between "self" and "non-self," but in certain individuals the immune system breaks down and interprets certain host tissues as foreign, manufacturing antibodies against their own tissues. Antibodies that have the host's own proteins as their specific antigens are known as *autoantibodies.* If they attack joints, rheumatoid arthritis develops. If they attack medium-sized arteries, *polyarteritis nodosa,* a systemic vasculitis characterized by necrotizing inflammatory lesions develops, and if they attack the thyroid, Graves' disease develops.

In autoimmune diseases the immune system is out of control. Powerful immune processes designed to defend the body become misdirected and attack host cells, tissues, and organs causing serious problems that are notoriously difficult to treat.

In early child development the infant's immune system learns to tolerate the proteins contained in food. These proteins are "foreign" but necessary, and the developing immune system learns not to react to them, a process known as *immune tolerance.* Most individuals develop such a tolerance to gluten proteins, but many never develop it and have a genetic susceptibility toward generating an immune response to gluten. The immune response against it sets off a chain reaction that develops into gluten intolerance, and eventually celiac disease.

Gluten and the Immune System: The Development of Gluten Intolerance and Celiac Disease

Gastroenterology is the study of diseases of the digestive system such as gastric ulcers, diverticulitis, and colorectal cancer.

Rheumatology is the study of diseases of the musculoskeletal system such as rheumatoid arthritis, lupus, gout, and ankylosing spondylitis.

A number of critical questions have puzzled researchers in the fields of gastroenterology, immunology, and rheumatology for many years.

- What is the nature of the immunological reaction to gluten?
- Why do people develop such profound symptoms and become sick as a result of eating foods containing wheat, barley, or rye?
- Why do only some of those genetically susceptible to developing gluten intolerance experience symptoms?
- Why might there be any relationship at all between gluten intolerance and autoimmune disorders?

These key questions have been investigated for decades, primarily in Europe, and many fascinating and complex answers have been provided. Immunology itself is a convoluted, intricate field. Immunologists investigating gluten intolerance have lost their way many times during the last 50 years, but persistence has yielded results and the last 20 years have seen successive breakthroughs.

Unlike other dietary proteins, gluten is not digestible by humans because our enzymes can only break gluten into large fragments. Some of these can be structurally transformed by a specific enzyme common to many locations throughout the body. One of these locations includes the cells within the lamina propria of the small intestine. In the past, celiac disease researchers have identified autoantibodies whose target was not specified. These autoantibodies were termed *antiendomysial antibodies* (AEA), which targeted an unknown protein found in the cells of the small intestinal lamina propria. After years of research, this protein was identified as the enzyme *tissue transglutaminase* (tTG), which was discussed at length in chapter two. The lamina propria, the small intestinal site of localization of tTG, is also the major site of immunological damage in celiac disease. The interaction of gluten fragments with tTG launches an immunological chain reaction.

The immunological background to this chain reaction is complicated. As discussed in chapter two, approximately 40% of individuals have a gene that leads to the construction of an immunologic tool known as HLA DQ2 or HLA DQ8. HLA stands for human leukocyte antigen, an antigen-displaying protein that is mounted like a flag on the surface of a white blood cell (leukocyte). HLA DQ2 is found in the majority of individuals with gluten intolerance and celiac disease. A related antigen-displaying protein, HLA DQ8, is found to a smaller extent in such individuals. HLA antigen-displaying proteins can lock onto and display your own (self) proteins, so other white blood cells (T cells) take notice of them. In this case, the signal means "do nothing, we're the good guys." Alternatively, antigen-displaying proteins can lock onto and display foreign (non-self) proteins. In that case, the signal means "send in the troops, these are bad guys."

HLA DQ2s and DQ8s don't normally interact with gluten fragments, but when the enzyme tTG changes a gluten fragment in the process of deamidation, the modified gluten protein structure causes it to be snatched up by HLA DQ2 and DQ8 antigen-displaying proteins. In a series of responses, your body reacts to the gluten proteins as a threat.

Unraveling this process identified a new mechanism in the development of autoimmunity. In their unmodified state, gluten proteins are tolerated by the immune system, but the actions of the enzyme tTG alter the gluten protein's structure, and this newly modified protein is recognized as foreign which sets off alarms. They interact with HLA DQ2 or DQ8 molecules, the HLA-antigen complex activates CD4+ T cells, and the immune response is off and running. In this way, enzyme-induced structural alterations create a "new" protein, which results in a process known as "breaking tolerance", ultimately creating autoantibodies.

How Does Gluten Launch an Autoimmune Response?

Cytokines are proteins that act as mediators of the immune response. They are signaling molecules that activate immunologic cells such as macrophages and natural killer cells. Cytokines are produced by lymphocytes, macrophages, NK cells, and some epithelial cells.

In a genetically susceptible individual, gluten can become an autoantigen. Its consumption can result in both innate and adaptive immune responses against this "foreign" protein. Regarding innate immunity, it is hypothesized that gluten proteins trigger a stress reaction in the epithelial cells lining the small intestine. These cells express the cytokine interleukin-15 (IL-15). IL-15 initiates two critical activities:

1. Increase in the numbers of intraepithelial lymphocytes (IELs) in the lamina propria (IEL expansion).
2. Increase in the numbers of natural killer receptors on the surface of the IELs (NK receptor expression).

IEL expansion and NK receptor expression causes the IELs to target and kill epithelial cells lining the inner wall of the small intestine, so the gluten-initiated innate immunity response acts to destroy the surface of the inner lining of the small intestine. These destructive changes frequently cause the characteristic symptoms of gluten intolerance and celiac disease: abdominal pain, abdominal bloating, diarrhea/constipation, and malabsorption syndrome.

Gluten also initiates an adaptive immunity response that begins with the transformation of gluten protein by tissue transglutaminase. The first question to discuss is how gluten proteins in the lumen of the small intestine come in contact with tTG, which is contained within certain cells in the lamina propria. Somehow these gluten fragments penetrate the epithelial barrier which is supposed to prevent foreign materials from gaining access to the cells and tissues of the host.

Environmental Triggers and Additional Genetic Factors

How do the gluten fragments reach these restricted areas? The answer demonstrates that genetics isn't the only factor causing a person to develop gluten intolerance. 40% of individuals have genes that code for HLA DQ2 or HLA DQ8, but only about 1% of the population has celiac disease. 1% instead 40% of people have celiac disease because an *environmental trigger* is necessary in addition to genetic predisposition.

Normally, foreign material is confined to the lumen of the gastrointestinal tract and is prevented from gaining access to the tissues comprising the wall of the tract. The primary barrier consists of the epithelial cells that form the innermost lining of the lumen and the *tight junctions* that cement these cells together. These tight junctions can become more permeable owing to a number of likely causes.

It is well known that both bacterial and viral infections cause immune responses and inflammatory reactions. A sufficiently extensive inflammatory reaction can break down structures in the small intestine, leading to increased permeability. Similarly, a sufficiently high fever can lead to increased gut permeability. Infection, inflammation, and wound healing may also cause the release of tTG from cells in the lamina propria. Increased gut permeability allows gluten protein fragments to come into contact with the now-available tTG. Another interesting theory suggests that gluten itself may rearrange tight junction proteins, resulting in increased permeability.

Environmental triggers including bacterial infection, viral infection, and fever may cause the protective barrier of the small intestine to become more permeable, allowing gluten peptides to gain access to the cells and tissues of the lamina propria. These environmental factors also cause cells in the lamina propria to release tTG. Next, through a complex series of metabolic and biochemical events, gluten causes an immunological response and an inflammatory reaction, leading to the signs and symptoms of gluten intolerance and celiac disease. It is also likely that additional inherited factors like genes coding for proteins that are not part of the HLA system are also involved in genetic susceptibility, but these genes have yet to be identified.

How Does a Person Become Susceptible?

As discussed, 40% of people have genes coding for HLA DQ2 and HLA DQ8 antigen-displaying proteins. These persons are genetically susceptible to gluten intolerance and celiac disease. In addition, all the other components in the gluten intolerance immune response, the tTG enzyme, HLA helper T cells, and B cells are present in all genetically susceptible individuals, but 1% rather than 40% develop celiac disease. Why do only a small portion of those who are genetically susceptible develop symptoms?

Two people can share an identical genetic sequence, but only one might demonstrate the specific characteristic encoded by that sequence. The expression of a genetic sequence, the manufacturing of a specific protein coded by that sequence, depends on a complex set of molecular factors. Usually there are a number of feedback mechanisms involved, some promoting, and others inhibiting gene expression and protein manufacture. The internal environment of the cell tips the balance in one direction or the other: gene expression or no gene expression. Person A and person B may have an identical genetic sequence and both may have sequences coding for antigen-presenting HLA DQ. but only person A will manufacture DQ2 or DQ8 proteins and develop gluten intolerance, all owing to person A's internal molecular environment.

In turn, a person's internal molecular environment depends to a large extent on his or her external environment, including diet. Studies demonstrate that people introduced to dietary gluten before the age of 4 months have a significantly higher risk of developing gluten intolerance and celiac disease. Additionally, bacterial infection, viral infection, and high fevers may all lead to increased permeability of the small intestine which could expose structures of the lamina propria to gluten proteins, setting off a cascade of immune responses that results in celiac disease.

Stress is another potential causative factor in the external environment. In one generalized model, ongoing stress often provokes an extended inflammatory reaction, which can stimulate an immunological response. If the gastrointestinal tract is involved, increased numbers of fibroblasts and macrophages lead to increased levels of tTG, increasing the likelihood of dietary gluten interacting with tTG, launching an immunological response that in the ongoing presence of dietary gluten, leads to gluten intolerance and celiac disease.

Not every person who has high levels of stress will develop gluten intolerance and celiac disease. Stress is one of many potential causative factors and in certain circumstances, stress may be an important contributor in the development of these problematic disorders.

When Gluten Meets tTG

Fibroblasts are cells that secrete materials used to support and stabilize the integrity of connective tissue, including bone, cartilage, and supporting layers of the lamina propria. Fibroblasts are the most common type of connective tissue cell.

tTG is found in many locations throughout the body. Various types of white blood cells, epithelial cells such as those lining the inner wall of the small intestine, and cells involved in wound healing such as fibroblasts are especially rich sources of tTG which catalyzes cross-linking reactions between protein molecules, connecting them with strong chemical bonds. These bonds are so strong that tTG has been described as nature's biological glue. tTG is normally stored inside cells and is released in response to various stresses.

A **substrate** is the molecule upon which an enzyme performs its actions. The substrate is transformed into a different molecule with different characteristics.

Enzymes are molecules that greatly increase the rate of biochemical reactions. Often, enzymes facilitate reactions that would not take place without their presence.

Amino acids are the molecular building blocks of proteins. Proteins in our food are digested in the gastrointestinal tract and broken down into their constituent amino acids. The amino acids cross the semipermeable small intestinal barrier and diffuse into the bloodstream where they are carried to various locations and used as raw materials for building new cells and tissues. Approximately 22 amino acids have been identified, including glutamine, proline, and glutamic acid.

Gluten is an excellent substrate for tTG activity owing to gluten's specific amino acid composition. If gluten is present, it is a preferential target for tTG which acts by deamidation of glutamine to glutamic acid. This process introduces a negative charge on the gluten molecules which increases the likelihood that gluten molecules will bind to HLA DQ2 or HLA DQ8 immunological proteins, launching an immunological reaction.

Where does this binding occur? HLA DQ2 and DQ8 proteins are embedded in the surfaces of *antigen-presenting cells,* (APCs), which are specialized immune cells, including dendritic cells and B lymphocytes that contain cell-surface receptors such as DQ2 and DQ8 that bind specific antigens (foreign proteins). DQ2 and DQ8 receptors preferentially bind to negatively charged molecules like gluten protein fragments.

Quick Recap

40% of Americans have the genetic capability to produce HLA DQ2 or DQ8 proteins and most Americans eat gluten containing breads and other foods. In a small proportion of them, the permeability of the small intestine can be compromised by infection, inflammation, or other trauma. In another small proportion, certain genes can cause susceptibility to a direct effect of gluten on small intestinal permeability.

Deamidation is a common process of protein modification in which one type of amino acid is converted into another. The process of deamidation introduces a negative charge on the protein structure. One function of deamidation may be to serve as a molecular clock and regulator of biological processes.

Dendritic cells are specialized cells of the immune system. They function as antigen-presenting cells. Dendritic cells have long, thin processes (dendrites) that capture foreign proteins and present these proteins to T lymphocytes. Dendritic cells help launch an immunological response to foreign proteins. They are found in many locations, including the lamina propria of the small intestine.

Infection, inflammation, or other trauma also releases tTG from epithelial cells, fibroblasts, and white blood cells contained within the lamina propria. Increased permeability allows gluten fragments to penetrate the lamina propria where they come in contact with tTG molecules. Gluten is a preferential substrate for tTG, and the enzyme deamidates these gluten fragments increasing gluten's binding capacity for DQ2 and DQ8 cell-surface receptors. When local antigen presenting cells containing DQ2 or DQ8 receptors latch onto gluten, the next phase of the immune response is launched.

APCs, T Cells, and B Cells

The language and notation describing immune system functioning are certainly complicated. Acronyms are frequently used for convenience to avoid restating the component's full name. The experience of encountering these complex explanations may be similar to being thrown into the deep end of the pool on your first day of learning how to swim. But the process is similar that involved in learning a foreign language. With a bit of concentration, things quickly become clear.

Immunological processes function through a complicated sequence of steps. When a foreign protein such as gluten is identified, certain specialized proteins such as HLA molecules recognize the antigen. Specialized cells (antigen-presenting cells) contain HLA molecules embedded in their surfaces. The HLA receptors capture specific antigens, then the APCs show the HLA-antigen complex to other specialized cells such as T cells.

APCs such as dendritic cells present the DQ–gluten complexes to specialized white blood cells known as CD4+ T cells. CD4 is a glycoprotein (a sugar–protein complex) expressed on the surface of certain T cells and CD4 is a co-receptor that assists T cells in recognizing antigens presented by APCs.

CD4+ T cells function as "helper" cells, acting as "middlemen" in another key component of the immunological response. After being activated by the gluten antigen, helper T cells activate another class of white blood cells known as B cells which produce antigen-specific antibodies, in this case antibodies to gluten protein fragments.

Helper T cells also assist other immunological cells in attacking, degrading, and destroying microorganisms and foreign proteins. Helper T cells are further subdivided into *Th1 cells* and *Th2 cells*. When Th1 and Th2 cells connect with APCs presenting DQ–gluten complexes they secrete *cytokines*, which stimulate additional immunological activities.

Cytokines are signaling molecules used in cellular communication. Some spur the growth of additional T cells and others attract specialized white blood cells to the local area of small intestine inflammation. These white blood cells, including *macrophages* and *neutrophils*, a type of phagocyte, participate in the inflammatory process. Cytokines signal macrophages to mobilize and kill invading cells and instruct macrophages to remove dead cells and various molecular bits and pieces.

Th1 cells express two potent cytokines — *tissue necrosis factor-a* (TNF-α) and *interferon-γ* (IFN-γ). TNF-α has many functions including inducing inflammation, inducing cell death, and inhibiting tumor growth. When TNF-α is produced in excess, it can participate in causing cancer. IFN-γ is a potent signaling molecule that enhances immunological functioning of many white blood cells, such as promoting killer cell (NK cell) activities.

Tissue necrosis factor and interferon-γ have profound effects on the structure and permeability of the epithelial barrier of the small intestine. IFN-γ rearranges the protein structure of these epithelial cells and the tight junctions connecting them. TNF-α also disrupts tight junction structure and assists the actions of IFN-γ. Permeability is increased, as is exposure of the epithelium in the lamina propria to gluten, perpetuating the immune and inflammatory reactions.

Additionally, TNF-α stimulates fibroblasts to secrete *matrix metalloproteases*, enzymes that cause destruction of connective tissue and breakdown of the mucosa, the inner lining of the small intestine. This destructive transformation of the mucosa results in the characteristic biopsy findings observed in celiac disease. Pathologic changes in the mucosa include the following:

- Crypt hyperplasia
- Intraepithelial lymphocytosis
- Villous atrophy

The **intestinal villi** are delicate fingerlike projections of the epithelial lining cells that extend into the intestinal lumen and exponentially increase the surface area available for the process of digestion.

The **crypts of Lieberkuhn** are depressions or crevices in between the villi. Epithelial cells lining the crypts are primarily involved in secretion of digestive enzymes. The bases of the crypts are lined by stem cells that develop into specialized epithelial cells.

In the destructive transformation of the mucosa, intestinal villi are eroded and become flattened. Crypts become enlarged in response to destruction of the villi. Large numbers of lymphocytes migrate to the area in response to the inflammatory processes. One significant result of villous atrophy is the loss of many digestive functions, which leads to malabsorption syndrome. All of these changes are initiated by the responses of Th1 helper T cells which are launched into action by recognizing the gluten antigen presented by antigen presenting cells containing the HLA DQ2 or DQ8 protein.

Activated Th2 helper T cells stimulate B lymphocytes to produce antibodies against gluten, perpetuating the immune response. Additionally, an immunological model of celiac disease suggests that B lymphocytes may themselves act as antigen presenting cells. These B cells bind tTG or tTG–gluten complexes and present the antigens to CD4+ T cells which secrete cytokines, causing proliferation of B cells that specifically produce *autoantibodies* to tTG.

As discussed, autoantibodies are antibodies that target your body's own proteins. At the beginning of the inflammatory/immunological cascade, tTG not only deamidates gluten protein fragments, but it can combine with the altered fragments to form new protein complexes. The tTG–gluten combination is known as a novel *epitope* (a large molecule that is recognized by the immune system). Helper T cells present the tTG–gluten epitope to certain B cells, that manufacture autoantibodies against tTG, known as anti-tTG. Identifying the presence of anti-tTG has become one of the gold standards in diagnosing celiac disease.

In gluten intolerance and celiac disease, antigen-presenting cells containing the molecular complex of HLA DQ2/DQ8 plus deamidated gluten cause CD4+ T cells to react. Th1 helper T cells launch a destructive inflammatory attack on the small intestinal mucosa and Th2 helper T cells stimulate B cells to produce antibodies to the foreign protein, gluten. B lymphocytes, through a complex interactive loop, produce antibodies to the body's own enzyme, tTG, increasing the strength and severity of the immune response, and as tTG is found in cells distributed widely throughout the body, the antibodies produced in celiac disease can cause autoimmune disorders that involve numerous tissues and organ systems.

Action Steps for Prevention and Treatment

Gluten-containing foods are staples in the Western diet and gluten is present in many household items and products. Should people change their lifestyles and take actions to avoid gluten on a daily basis? For those not susceptible, the short answer is no, but on the other hand, knowledge is power.

First-degree relatives, parents, siblings, and children of people with gluten intolerance are at increased risk. These relatives of individuals with gluten intolerance or celiac disease could be tested for the presence of anti-tTG autoantibody. This test is highly specific and a positive test for anti-tTG autoantibody strongly suggests the presence of gluten intolerance and celiac disease, with or without symptoms.

Furthermore, persons with type 1 diabetes or other autoimmune diseases are at increased risk of developing celiac disease. Gluten intolerance and celiac disease may be present in children with

ADHD, autism, and other neuropsychiatric disorders. Persons with schizophrenia may also have undiagnosed celiac disease. Additionally, gluten intolerance and celiac disease may be implicated in infertility and cases of multiple miscarriages and people with a gastrointestinal tract malignancy may have co-existing celiac disease. Screening these at-risk individuals represents an important public health initiative. People with any of these disorders or parents of affected children can be proactive and take action on their own behalf. A blood test will indicate whether further steps are needed.

Infants and young children with chronic abdominal pain, abdominal bloating, and diarrhea/constipation should be tested for anti-tTG autoantibody. Similarly, children failing to thrive and those in whom malabsorption syndrome is suspected should be tested for anti-tTG autoantibody.

People who may have undiagnosed gluten intolerance and celiac disease include those, young and old, with osteoporosis, as well as those with endocrine diseases affecting the thyroid or adrenal glands. Anti-tTG autoantibody testing will facilitate the diagnosis of co-existing celiac disease.

Early diagnosis can help avoid years of suffering and help prevent the development of serious co-morbidities such as malignancy and various autoimmune diseases. The best public health strategy is to avoid introducing gluten-containing foods in a newborn's diet until the infant is six months old. After six months, slowly adding such foods to the child's diet will help establish immune tolerance. Adding an overwhelming quantity of gluten-containing foods to any young person's diet can lead to gluten intolerance and celiac disease.

For those responsible for their own health, older teenagers and adults, knowledge is power. Persistent signs and symptoms require thorough investigation. The key is to pay attention and listen to your body. Pain usually means something is wrong, unless you can specifically account for the presence of that particular pain (as in the case of an exercise or sports-related injury). We're not going to run to the doctor whenever we experience a new pain, but pain that lingers needs to be evaluated. Additionally, pain and other signs and symptoms that do not get better with treatment need to be reevaluated. New causes and new diagnoses need to be considered. There may not be a need for extensive new tests, but there is a need for new thinking, meaning reassessment of the clinical circumstances and potential etiologies. Gluten intolerance and celiac disease may be at the root of a wide variety of conditions and need to be considered on a day-to-day basis, not only by physicians, but by any person with an unexpected and unexplained medical situation.

Leaky Gut Syndrome

I'm Gluten-Free Why Don't I Feel Better?

Jennifer Walker's medical travails began with an unsettling skin disorder in March 2010. The fit 40-year-old had previously never suffered from hives until these blotches appeared on her face and arms, then her head, torso, and legs. Jennifer consulted with three dermatologists in April 2010, all of whom wanted to prescribe Prednisone, but none of these specialists could formulate a diagnosis or ascertain a cause for Jennifer's symptoms. She also saw two rheumatologists in June and July, but Jennifer said they "basically sent me away" without identifying any cause of her skin problem. She continued taking Prednisone intermittently for pain relief and sleep, but she didn't improve and didn't wish to take such strong medication long-term.

Following a difficult and stressful summer, she had lunch with a friend who was being treated in our clinic and described us as "detectives." Jennifer's friend was adamant that she see us right away, but instead, Jennifer and her husband took a seven day cruise. While onboard she ate an abundance of cookies, bread, pasta, and sauces. In other words, she ate "as much gluten as you possibly can." Soon after the cruise, her rash became worse and Jennifer couldn't get out of bed. She described the full-blown rash as "raw" and "awful", so she "pretty much stopped eating" and lost ten pounds, representing 10% of her prior weight of 100 pounds. Her hair was falling out in chunks and she lost 90% of it. She couldn't sleep and "couldn't formulate a sentence." Only able to sleep 1 or 2 hours a night, she soon became physically exhausted.

Jennifer recalled her friend's recommendation and met with us in December 2010. After initial consultation and lab tests, we recommended a gluten and dairy free diet. The immediate result was that the more she ate certain foods, the more she became allergic to them and was down to ten foods she could eat. We also recommended a course of probiotic food supplements. As a result of her gluten and diary-free diet, she regained the ten pounds she had lost, her hair grew back to normal, and her brain fog and fatigue resolved, but Jennifer continued to respond adversely to gluten in her environment.

"I was 100% gluten free but continued to have problems once a month." When that occurred, "I would be down for ten days." We concluded the cause was airborne gluten particles. When Jennifer encountered them in a store or in a relative's home, her rash reappeared, her brain fogged, and she would be bedridden for more than a week. Shopping at Costco, visiting the local supermarket, or going into any bakery triggered severe symptoms within 24 hours. She became sick merely by entering a restaurant or any home where gluten containing foods were being prepared. "Breathing gluten" was a serious problem that needed to be addressed.

Ultimately, Jennifer modified her habits. "We used to eat out almost every day, sometimes twice a day," she said. Now she cooks at home and brings her own food when she and her husband visit friends and family. She also calls in advance and inquires whether her hosts have done any baking within the prior 48 hours. If baking is required, Jennifer asks if it can take place outside the house until the ingredients are wet. Her family and friends are glad to accommodate her requests.

It took three years for her to achieve a substantial recovery and Dr. Shikhman's identification of airborne gluten as a hidden source of toxicity was a key component of her return to good health.

"Dr. Shikhman never gives up. He's a detective and tells you he will find your problem," she said. "I've figured out how to live my life in an absolutely different way. I'm learning."

Gastrointestinal Tract Permeability

The gastrointestinal tract is described as the largest surface of the human body in contact with the external environment. The epithelial barrier of the small intestine covers an area of approximately 250 to 400 square meters. At the mucosal surface, the intestinal epithelial barrier separates billions of bacteria and viruses from the lamina propria, the site of the largest segment of our body's immune system. An intact and functioning barrier protects against invasion by microorganisms and toxins. Conversely, the intestinal epithelial barrier must be open to permit absorption of essential nutrients and fluids. Specific adaptations of the intestinal mucosa permit interactions with the commensal microbiota without eliciting chronic inflammation, while providing an appropriate inflammatory response to a threat from pathogenic microorganisms.

The intestinal epithelial barrier consists of a physical barrier and a chemical barrier. The physical barrier is composed of epithelial cells and a gel layer formed by various epithelial mucosal secretions. The chemical barrier consists of antimicrobial peptides, cytokines, other inflammatory mediators, and digestive secretions. A central regulator of the intestinal epithelial barrier is the intestinal microbiota.

An effective barrier to foreign pathogens and antigens is critical for optimum functioning of the gut and the health and well-being of the organism as a whole. Tight junction proteins critical for determining intestinal epithelial permeability are composed of complex protein systems that are organized by transmembrane proteins (occludin and the claudin family) interacting with intracellular zonula occludens proteins that bind to the actin cytoskeleton architecture, an elaborate network of protein filaments that extends throughout the gel-like cytoplasm. It is essential for maintaining cellular structure. Zonula occludens proteins are scaffolding proteins that provide a structural framework for assembly of protein complexes at the cytoplasmic surface of intercellular junctions. When actin contracts, paracellular permeability to small molecules and electrolytes is increased.

Tight junction structure and function are influenced by a diversity of physiological and pathological stimuli such as luminal glucose which causes increased intestinal epithelial permeability to small molecules. Cytokines and macrophages in the epithelial region also regulate intestinal epithelial permeability by impacting the tight junction protein complex and the actin cytoskeleton. As an example of pathology, in celiac disease the intestinal epithelial barrier is compromised by decreased expression and altered distribution of tight junction proteins.

Overall, disruption of the intestinal epithelial barrier leads to increased intestinal permeability (leaky gut syndrome) as well as *dysbiosis*, a microbial imbalance that causes alterations in composition or function of the usual microbiome. In leaky gut syndrome, various commensal and pathogenic microorganisms cross the barrier and contact inflammatory cells residing in the lamina propria, initiating an inflammatory response.

What is Leaky Gut Syndrome?

Leaky gut syndrome is a highly-defined functional disorder of the gastrointestinal tract resulting from abnormal intestinal permeability. A primary function of the intestinal epithelial lining is to establish selective intestinal permeability through tight junctions between adjacent epithelial mucosal cells. Disruption of the tight junction structure results in increased intestinal permeability; hence the term "leaky gut syndrome". In a healthy intestinal tract with intact tight junctions, the mucosal membrane allows nutrients to pass the barrier and blocks entry of toxins and pathogens to the bloodstream. In unhealthy intestinal tracts the tight junction structure becomes loose, increasing intestinal mucosal permeability, allowing pathogens into the bloodstream. The "tightness" of tight junctions is regulated by zonulin, a protein that maintains the integrity of tight junction structure. Research has demonstrated that production and release of zonulin is increased by gluten, which causes "leakiness" of the intestinal epithelial mucosa. Zonulin overexpression leads to loosening of the tight junction structure, increasing intestinal mucosal permeability.

The degree of leakage can be objectively measured and monitored with two specific groups of laboratory tests. The first measures the concentration of zonulin in the blood. Elevated zonulin indicates the presence of leaky gut syndrome. The second group of tests measures the ability of non-digested sugar molecules such as lactulose to be absorbed through the intestinal mucosa and enter the bloodstream. To perform this test, the patient drinks a lactulose solution. Elevated urine lactulose levels indicates the presence of leaky gut syndrome.

With disruption of tight junctions and resultant leaky gut syndrome, the intestinal mucosal membrane is inflamed, irritated, and compromised. Intestinal barrier dysfunction and damage to intestinal villi interfere with nutrient absorption, while permitting toxins, pathogens, and antigen–antibody complexes to enter the bloodstream. Circulating immune complexes cause systemic inflammation, autoimmune responses, additional malabsorption, and nutrient deficiency. Further, circulating immune complexes can breach the blood–brain barrier with resultant neuropsychiatric symptoms and disorders such as autism, multiple sclerosis, and schizophrenia.

Common causes of leaky gut syndrome include:

- Chemotherapy
- Chronic use of alcohol
- Chronic use of corticosteroid medications such as prednisone, methylprednisone, and hydrocortisone
- Chronic use of estrogen-containing medications such as birth control pills and medications provided as hormone replacement therapy
- Chronic use of nonsteroidal anti-inflammatory drugs such as ibuprofen, naproxen, and diclofenac
- Chronic yeast (Candida) infection
- Diet containing excessive carbohydrates or other imbalances
- Imbalance between beneficial and pathogenic intestinal microorganisms (dysbiosis)
- Intestinal parasite infection
- Prolonged use of antibiotics
- Radiation therapy

Triggers causing intestinal damage with resultant leaky gut syndrome include dietary proteins such as gluten, low gastric hydrochloric acid, low gastric enzymes, infections, blood sugar issues, food allergies, exposure to toxins, pregnancy, menopause, and stress.

Symptoms of leaky gut syndrome include:

- Abdominal bloating and discomfort after eating
- Acne, hives, and eczema
- Brain fog
- Diarrhea
- Fatigue, muscle weakness, and muscle pain associated with eating
- Food-associated headaches
- Mucus in the stool
- Poor tolerance of alcohol

Leaky gut syndrome is associated with various diseases and disorders including:

- Ankylosing spondylitis
- Asthma
- Autoimmune hepatitis
- Chronic fatigue
- Chronic sinusitis
- Type 1 Diabetes
- Eczema
- Hay fever
- Increased symptoms of celiac disease and gluten intolerance
- Increased symptoms of ulcerative colitis or Crohn's disease
- Migraine headaches
- Psoriasis and psoriatic arthritis
- Rheumatoid arthritis

Treatment of Leaky Gut Syndrome

Treatment of leaky gut syndrome includes:

- Eliminating immunogenic foods
- Eliminating potential triggers such as alcohol, antibiotics, and NSAIDs
- Improving digestion

- Normalizing the intestinal microbiome
- Optimizing diet
- Optimizing the intestinal epithelial mucosal immune responses
- Repairing and restoring tight junctions

Detection of immunogenic foods is based on food intolerance testing and may investigate leukocyte (white blood cell) activation by the putative immunogenic food. Other tests are based on measuring antibody levels in blood or saliva in response to specific foods. Clinical experience demonstrates that IgG_4-based food intolerance testing is highly correlated with positive responses to the food elimination diet.

In addition to elimination of gluten and cross-reactive foods, diet optimization typically involves reduction of carbohydrate consumption, elimination of spicy foods, and increased consumption of foods with high fiber concentrations and fermented foods. Optimal results are achieved on the basis of a highly individualized diet utilizing food intolerance test results.

Improved digestion is accomplished with supplementation utilizing various digestive enzymes, ox bile, and milk thistle.

Normalizing the intestinal microbiome is accomplished by supplementation with high-dose probiotics (greater than 100 billion CFU [colony-forming units] per day) and prebiotics. Probiotics used in the treatment of leaky gut syndrome include GoldenBiotic-8, *Saccharomyces boulardii*, and *Bacillus coagulans*. Prebiotics used in the treatment of leaky gut syndrome include Psyllium/Apple Pectin, Mannan Oligosaccharides, Glucomannan, and Galactooligosaccharides. Mannan Oligosaccharides act to detach harmful microorganisms such as Shigella, Salmonella, and Candida from the intestinal wall.

Mannan Oligosaccharides assist in repairing intestinal villi structure and restoring normal intestinal mucosal permeability. Galactooligosaccharides are a strong stimulant to growth of beneficial intestinal bacteria such as lactobacilli and bifidobacteria. Galactooligosaccharides also stimulate differentiation and development of natural killer cells, which protect the body from infection.

Intestinal mucosal immune responses are optimized by

supplementation with immunobiotics such as Mannan Oligosaccharides; stimulants of mucosal immune responses such as Epicor and Bovine Immunoglobulins, Black Currant Seed Oil, and activators of natural killer cells such as Coix Seed Extract, Beta-Glucan/Arabinogalactan, and Cordyceps Sinensis, a medicinal mushroom. Repair and restoration of tight junctions is accomplished by supplementation with Leaky Gut Aid Day, Leaky Gut Aid Night, N-Acetylcysteine, and N-Acetyl Glucosamine. Leaky Gut Aid formulations consist of calcium and magnesium salts of butyric acid. Tight junctions are restored and repaired by supplementation with salts of butyric acid. In the intestine, butyrate salts act to regulate intestinal permeability and fluid transport, modulate immune and inflammatory responses, and optimize intestinal transit time. Additionally, butyrate salts suppress Candida overgrowth. Supplementation with butyrate salts effectively treats leaky gut syndrome through repair of tight junctions and restoration of intestinal permeability.

Leaky Gut Syndrome, Celiac Disease, and Other Autoimmune Disorders

The intestinal epithelium provides an interface between the external environment and the host and coordinates digestive, absorptive, and immunological functions. Additionally, it regulates molecular trafficking between the intestinal lumen, the lamina propria, and the bloodstream through the paracellular space (the interstices between intestinal epithelial cells). Permeability of large molecules is regulated by the configuration of intercellular tight junctions. Alterations in tight junction competency are associated with the development of autoimmune diseases.

The combination of three pre-existing conditions leads to an autoimmune response. The first is the genetic susceptibility of the person's immune system to recognize, and possibly misinterpret an environmental antigen such as gluten proteins present within the intestinal lumen. The second condition is exposure of the host to the antigen. Third, the antigen must be presented to the intestinal mucosal immune system located in the lamina propria.

Normally, such paracellular passage is prevented by competent tight junctions, but their disruption leads to increased intestinal epithelial permeability, resulting in an abnormality of antigen delivery. The continuous stimulation of the immune system by "non-self" antigens (environmental triggers) results in "molecular mimicry," in which an immune response is launched against "self" antigens that resemble the "non-self" antigens. This miscommunication causes a multi-organ autoimmune response which can be halted if the ongoing exposure to environmental triggers is eliminated.

The pathophysiology of celiac disease exemplifies this autoimmune pathway. Patients with celiac disease typically demonstrate genetic susceptibility in the form of human leukocyte antigen (HLA) genes, including HLA DQ2 and DQ8. There is a highly specific autoimmune response to tissue transglutaminase autoantigen. The environmental trigger is gliadin, a large protein fragment derived from the partial digestion of gluten. Normally, the interaction between HLAs and gluten is prevented by intact intestinal epithelial tight junctions, but early in celiac disease, tight junction structure is disrupted. By employing a strict gluten free diet, symptoms resolve, concentrations of proinflammatory cytokines return to normal, and autoimmune damage to the intestinal epithelium is repaired. These findings provide evidence that an autoimmune process can be reversed if environmental triggers like gluten can be eliminated, permitting normalization of intestinal epithelial barrier function.

Tight junctions must be capable of dynamic and coordinated responses to diverse physiological challenges. Research has demonstrated that the zonulin system appears to reversibly regulate intestinal permeability and movement of macromolecules, white blood cells, and fluid between the intestinal lumen and the bloodstream. The zonulin system accomplishes these changes by modulating tight junction structure and function. Zonulin release is triggered by exposure of the intestinal epithelium to gluten and various bacteria.

The chemokine receptor CXCR3 has been identified as the target intestinal receptor for gliadin. The binding of gliadin to CXCR3 is critical for zonulin release and the resulting increase in intestinal epithelial permeability. Zonulin overexpression has been demonstrated in patients with celiac disease and patients with type 1 diabetes. In a recent study, 81% of 190 celiac disease patients and 50% of their first-degree relatives had serum zonulin levels two standard deviations above the mean for age-matched healthy controls. In comparison, only 4.9% of 101 controls had zonulin levels two standard deviations above the mean. Similarly, 42% of 339 patients with type 1 diabetes and 29% of their first-degree relatives had serum zonulin levels two standard deviations above the mean for age-matched healthy controls. In comparison, only 4% of 97 controls had zonulin levels two standard deviations above the mean.

Probiotics and Treatment of Leaky Gut Syndrome

Alterations in the intestinal epithelial barrier and increased intestinal permeability are associated with numerous intestinal and systemic diseases including celiac disease, ulcerative colitis, irritable bowel syndrome, autoimmune diseases such as rheumatoid arthritis, obesity, and metabolic diseases. In addition to dietary factors, viral intestinal infections, environmental toxins, and chronic inflammation play a role in disruption of intestinal epithelial tight junctions. These barrier defects are related to increased activity of proinflammatory cytokines such as TNF-α, interleukin-Iβ, and interleukin-13, which are elevated in the chronically inflamed intestine. Intestinal barrier dysfunction is a primary feature of celiac disease and inflammatory bowel disease.

Probiotics are frequently used in the treatment of leaky gut syndrome and other gastrointestinal disorders involving disruption of the intestinal epithelial barrier. Probiotics act through restoration of tight junction integrity and homeostasis with respect to intestinal permeability. A specific probiotic, *L. rhamnosus GG*, accelerates the maturation of the intestinal epithelial barrier. One study investigated treatment with probiotics in children with increased intestinal permeability and atopic dermatitis. In this double-blind, placebo-controlled trial, a mixture of two probiotics, *L. rhamnosus* and *L. reuteri*, was administered for six weeks to 41 children. Following treatment, a significant reduction in intestinal permeability was detected. Probiotics have been characterized as live microbial supplements that beneficially affect the patient by improving intestinal microbial balance. Numerous studies report that probiotics promote integrity of the intestinal epithelial barrier.

> **Prebiotics** are non-digestible carbohydrate-based food ingredients that stimulate the growth of beneficial bacteria (bifidobacteria and lactic acid bacteria) in the gastrointestinal tract.

Research suggests that probiotics and prebiotics have beneficial effects in leaky gut syndrome, chronic inflammatory disease, and metabolic disorders. In addition to going on and maintaining a gluten-free diet, patients with gluten intolerance and associated leaky gut syndrome can benefit from prebiotics and probiotics which assist in improving intestinal epithelial barrier function and reconstituting the commensal microbiota. The likely result is amelioration of chronic inflammatory changes, reduction in symptoms, and a return to good health.

Leaky Gut Syndrome Self-Assessment

Based on what we see in our practice and what we know about Leaky Gut Syndrome, answering yes to the following questions are good indicators that you may have Leaky Gut.

1. Do you experience fatigue after eating?

2. Can you tolerate alcohol?

3. Do you frequently use NSAIDs such as ibuprofen, naproxen, and diclofenac?

4. Do you frequently use antibiotics?

5. Do you experience abdominal discomfort and bloating?

6. Do you experience frequent yeast infections?

7. Do you experience frequent diarrhea?

8. Do you experience frequent migraine headaches?

9. Do you have multiple food allergies?

10. Do you have eczema?

For more in depth results please take our online self-assessment at: glutenfreeremedies.com

Scoring

Low Probability (less than 20%): 1-2 questions

Moderate Probability (50/50 chance): 3-4 questions

High Probability (over 75%): over 4 questions

Specific supplements can be helpful, based upon indicated symptoms:

1. If you experience fatigue after eating: Vegan Digestive Enzymes, Leaky Gut Aid, and Leaky Gut Probiotic

2. If you frequently use NSAIDs: Leaky Gut Aid

3. If you frequently use antibiotics: *Bacillus coagulans*, GoldenBiotic-8, Leaky Gut Aid, and Mannan Oligosaccharides

4. If you experience abdominal discomfort and bloating: Leaky Gut Aid, Leaky Gut Probiotic, Vegan Digestive Enzymes, and Triphala

5. If you experience frequent yeast infections: Leaky Gut Aid, Leaky Gut Probiotic, Berberine, Pau D'Arco, Black Walnut Hulls, GoldenBiotic-8, and Mannan Oligosaccharides

6. If you experience frequent diarrhea: Leaky Gut Aid, Leaky Gut Probiotic, and GoldenBiotic-8

7. If you experience frequent migraine headaches: Butterbur/Feverfew Blend

8. If you have eczema: GoldenBiotic-8, *Bacillus coagulans*, Leaky Gut Probiotic, and Plant Digestive Enzymes may be helpful.

Additional Technical Reading

The information in this section is very scientific, and while important, is not compatible with the style of the rest of the book. For those who require a deeper dive into the science behind Leaky Gut Syndrome, read on.

The Intestinal Epithelial Barrier

The intestinal epithelium (the outermost layer of cells lining the gastrointestinal tract) is a barrier composed of a single layer of cells with a thickness of only 20 microns (a micron is one-millionth of a meter). This single-cell layer is all that separates the contents of the intestinal lumen from reactive immune cells residing in the lamina propria, the highly vascular layer of connective tissue underlying the intestinal epithelial cells. Within the lamina propria, a complex network of immune cells is organized into *gut-associated lymphoid tissue* (GALT) which contains approximately 70% of the body's immune cells. It is responsible for immune tolerance of the commensal microbiota (the 100 trillion non-pathogenic microorganisms residing in the gut) and the immune response to pathogenic microorganisms. The lamina propria together with the epithelium constitute the intestinal mucosa.

Intestinal permeability is the property of the intestinal epithelium that allows dissolved molecules and fluids to be exchanged between the intestinal lumen, the intestinal mucosa, and the bloodstream. A key function of the intestinal epithelium enables nutrients to diffuse across the barrier, but prevents its permeation by molecules that cause inflammation (proinflammatory molecules) such as antigens (foreign proteins), toxins, and pathogenic microorganisms. Alteration or disruption of the intestinal epithelial barrier permits leakage of the luminal contents to the underlying mucosal tissues and into the bloodstream resulting in activation of the immune response and generation of intestinal inflammation. This alteration in permeability is implicated in the pathogenesis of many diseases, including celiac disease, inflammatory bowel disease, and autoimmune disorders.

Simple columnar epithelial cells demonstrate physical and biochemical adaptations to maintain integrity of the barrier. These include epithelial tight junctions, secreted mucinous proteins that attach to the luminal border of the epithelial cells, and production of numerous antimicrobial peptides. Specialized dendritic cells can extend in branch-like extensions between tight junctions to sample luminal contents.

The intestinal epithelial tight junctions are protein complexes that form a selectively permeable seal between adjoining epithelial cells lining the intestinal lumen. The interaction of the protein complexes dictates the competency of the tight junctions. Tight junction barrier function and permeability between cells is regulated by numerous stimuli and is directly associated with our overall health and susceptibility to disease. Disruption of this barrier leads to increased permeability, followed by translocation of proinflammatory molecules and microorganisms to the intestinal epithelium and activation of the immune system of the intestinal mucosa. The result is sustained inflammatory changes and tissue damage. Barrier defects are identified in a variety of gastrointestinal diseases including celiac disease and Crohn's disease, as well as in systemic diseases like rheumatoid arthritis and multiple sclerosis. In extreme circumstances, compromised intestinal barrier function can lead to a whole body inflammatory state and multiple organ failure.

Tight junctions are composed of more than 50 proteins. Multiple protein complexes connect intestinal epithelial cells at their upper and inner margins. Transmembrane proteins seal the paracellular space between epithelial cells and mediate cell-to-cell adhesion. Transmembrane proteins also extend across the cellular plasma membrane and interact with the actin cytoskeleton within the epithelial cell. Four such transmembrane proteins have been identified, including *occludin* and the *claudin* family.

Tight junction proteins have intracellular components, domains that reside within the cytoplasm of adjacent cells. These intracellular domains connect with scaffolding proteins such as zonula occludens proteins which anchor the transmembrane proteins to intracellular cytoskeleton proteins. The overall structure created by these complex interactions is exceedingly stable and dynamically permeable. A belt-like structure encircles the upper pole of intestinal epithelial cells and projects *actin filaments* that interface with tight junction proteins. Circumferential contractions of this ring regulate tight junction configuration and intestinal epithelial permeability. As a result, permeability of the intestinal barrier changes in response to the state of the host and the constitution of the luminal environment. Such factors include heredity, stress, diet, intestinal microorganisms, infectious agents, drugs, and toxins. Tight junctions are constantly being remodeled owing to interactions with various external stimuli, including commensal microorganisms and pathogenic bacteria.

The transmembrane protein occludin participates in assembly and maintenance of tight junctions. The interactions of the claudin proteins create barriers against or openings for the passage of selected molecules. The *zonula occludens* proteins were the first tight junction proteins to be identified. They provide intracellular scaffolding support to tight junctions and are necessary for maintenance and regulation of tight junction structure. Tight junction proteins also participate in developmental, physiological, and pathological processes, and the movement of macromolecules, fluids, and white blood cells from the intestinal lumen to the bloodstream and vice versa. In association with lymphoid tissue residing in the gut (Peyer's patches), and the neuroendocrine network, the intestinal epithelium helps maintain equilibrium in the immune response to non-self antigens. Compromise of tight junction function leads to penetration of the intestinal epithelial barrier by foreign immunogenic antigens, contact with the lamina propria by these antigens, initiation of an inflammatory cascade, and subsequent development of autoimmune disease such as autoimmune thyroiditis, celiac disease, rheumatoid arthritis, and type 1 diabetes.

The tight junction barrier can break down owing to a local inflammatory process. The immediate causes of such tight junction disruption are inflammatory cytokines including interferon-γ, tumor necrosis factor-α, interleukin-Iβ, and interleukin-17. Cytokines are cell signaling molecules that facilitate cell-to-cell communication in immune responses. These chemical messengers are also known as immunomodulating agents that participate in modulating an immune response. Tight junction barrier dysfunction resulting from contact with proinflammatory cytokines leads to activation of the immune system and tissue inflammation. Such responses are associated with the initiation or development of numerous intestinal and systemic diseases.

Interferon-γ (IFN-γ) actions include rearranging the infracellular protein cytoskeleton and redistributing tight junction proteins resulting in disruption of the tight junction and increased permeability between intestinal epithelial cells. Tumor necrosis factor-α (TNF-α) is produced by activated T cells and macrophages, (white blood cells that function in the immune response.) TNF-α provokes an inflammatory response in intestinal epithelial cells and causes tight junction dysfunction. Interleukin-Iβ levels are elevated in the intestinal epithelium in inflammatory diseases such as celiac disease. Interleukin-Iβ causes impaired tight junction function with increased permeability. Interleukin-17, a cytokine produced by Th17 cells (a subset of helper T cells), is a potent inducer of tissue inflammation. Interleukin-17 is associated with the development of numerous autoimmune diseases including inflammatory bowel diseases, celiac disease, rheumatoid arthritis, and multiple sclerosis. Autoimmune diseases affect as many as 24 million people in the United States, representing approximately 8% of the population.

Inflammatory bowel diseases, including Crohn's disease and ulcerative colitis, represent a continuum of disorders. Research has demonstrated that levels of inflammatory cytokines such as interferon-γ, tumor necrosis factor-α, and interleukin-17 are increased in the intestinal epithelium of patients with celiac disease and inflammatory bowel disease. These proinflammatory molecules are implicated in disruption of tight junction function. Increased intestinal permeability caused by tight junction dysfunction is a feature common to these conditions and other inflammatory diseases, so dynamic regulation by cytokines of the intestinal tight junction barrier is a key component of the pathogenesis of many inflammatory diseases.

The intestinal epithelial barrier and associated tight junctions controls the balance between tolerance of and immunity to antigens identified as non-self. Tight junction dysfunction can disrupt this equlibrium, shifting the balance toward an immune response and development of autoimmune disease. Tight junction leakage is promoted by various dietary factors, including gluten, dairy, legumes, starchy vegetables, sugar, alcohol, spicy food, grains, and high glycemic fruits. This leakage permits foreign antigens to penetrate the intestinal epithelial barrier and initiate or perpetuate an immune reaction, possibly activating an autoimmune cascade.

When the protection provided by the intestinal epithelial barrier is disrupted, antigens in the intestinal lumen come into direct contact with immune cells in the lamina propria resulting in impairment of normal barrier functions such as the recognition of "self" antigens and tolerance toward the intestinal microbiota. A vicious circle is established in which proinflammatory cytokines such as TNF-α and IFN- γ disrupt tight junction structure, leading to alteration in intestinal epithelial permeability. Contact of translocated luminal contents with immune cells in the lamina propria leads to an immune response, generating increased levels of proinflammatory cytokines. Further tight junction modification perpetuates the vicious loop and an increasingly destructive response.

The prevalence of autoimmune diseases such as celiac disease, lupus, rheumatoid arthritis, autoimmune thyroiditis, and type 1 diabetes is increasing throughout westernized societies. The omnipresence of gluten in westernized diets is a significant factor and it is well known that gluten is the causative agent in celiac disease. Research has demonstrated that tissue transglutaminase is the specific autoantigen precipitating the immune response that results in celiac disease. Studies show that gluten's main antigen, gliadin, causes a rearrangement of the zonulin transmembrane proteins and resultant compromise of tight junction competence indicating that gluten is directly responsible for increased intestinal epithelial permeability in celiac disease. The abnormally increased permeability results in exposure of immune cells embedded in the intestinal epithelium to gliadin. Gliadin binding to T cell active sites incites an additional inflammatory cascade, further increasing intestinal epithelial permeability, creating a self-perpetuating positive feedback loop of inflammatory response. Overall, gluten is a multifactorial stimulator of the immune system with at least 50 toxic epitopes (the part of the antigen that is recognized by the immune system) in gluten peptides that have immunomodulatory and cytotoxic effects that act to permeate the intestinal epithelial barrier.

There is a significant association between gastrointestinal and systemic diseases and alterations in intestinal permeability. Research has consistently demonstrated that an increase in intestinal permeability (as in leaky gut syndrome) contributes to the exacerbation of gastrointestinal and systemic diseases. In many cases, treatment that leads to restoration of intestinal homeostasis also leads to reduction in or resolution of disease-related symptoms.

Intestinal Microorganisms

During gestation and after birth, human gastrointestinal tracts are colonized from the environment by a gradually increasing diversity and volume of bacteria, fungi, and viruses. A human body is colonized by more than 100 trillion commensal microorganisms termed microbiota. This microbiome contributes to the host's adaptation to the environment and modulates immune system activities so as not to reject these symbiotic fellow travelers. These microorganisms are involved in molecular "crosstalk" with the intestinal epithelium and impact intestinal epithelial barrier function. Several species of bacteria utilize various mechanisms and signaling pathways to regulate tight junction structure and function.

Intestinal microorganisms participate in the metabolism of nutrients and induce immunity. The microbiota is involved in the breakdown and absorption of nutrients, production of hormones and vitamins, and prevention of colonization by pathogenic microorganisms. Intestinal microorganisms can indirectly affect intestinal epithelial barrier function by fermenting undigested carbohydrates in the intestine. For example, the production of butyrate by bacteria in the large intestine enhances the small intestinal epithelial barrier by promoting tight junction assembly.

> **Probiotics** are live microbial supplements that beneficially affect the patient by improving intestinal microbial balance.

Probiotics such as *Lactobacilli* and *Bifidobacteria* produce bactericidal acidic molecules such as short-chain fatty acids (SCFAs) which participate in stimulating mucus production, blocking invasion and adherence of the pathogen *Escherichia coli*, and increasing total and pathogen-specific immunoglobulin A in the mucosa.

> **Homeostasis** is the tendency of the body to seek and maintain a condition of balance or equilibrium within its internal environment, even when faced with external changes.

The intestinal microbiota produce nutrients used by epithelial mucosal cells and their composition and diversity participate in balancing inflammatory and tolerance responses of the immune system. They play a critical role in maintaining intestinal homeostasis. Changes in composition of the microorganisms inhabiting the intestinal tract is likely involved in disruption of tight junction protein structure and decreased manufacture of these transmembrane proteins, so alterations in the intestinal microbiome are associated with the development of intestinal disorders and systemic diseases such as celiac disease, cancer, obesity, type 1 diabetes, and neuropathological disorders like autism and depression. Many of these diseases are associated with altered intestinal epithelial barrier function and increased permeability known as leaky gut syndrome.

It is well established that host adaptation is influenced by the microbiome which adds new genes and capabilities that promote increased flexibility in one's diet. Commensal microorganisms influence the host's intestinal immune response as is the case when the microbiota participate in development of Peyer's patches. Certain components of the intestinal microbiota can induce specific responses of the immune system such as immunoglobulin A (IgA) mediated responses and development of Th1/Th17 helper T cells and regulatory T cells. Th17 cell development depends on the presence of commensal microorganisms and dietary antigens and improve intestinal epithelial barrier function by stimulating mucin production, increasing transport of IgA to the lumen, and enhancing function of tight junction proteins. IgA is the principal immunoglobulin of intestinal mucous secretions and has a central role in immune function and protection against pathogens. In a reflexive feedback loop, IgA provides homeostatic regulation of the intestinal microbiome and prevents mucosal inflammation by trapping antigens or pathogens in the mucosal layer (immune exclusion), removing antigen-antibody complexes in the lamina propria, and neutralizing inflammatory cytokines.

Overall, the intestinal immune system has to distinguish commensal from foreign (pathogenic) microorganisms. In a reflexive feedback loop, this sensing of commensals is critical for the development and effective functioning of the host immune system. The intestinal microbiota provide signals to induce healthy immune system development, stimulate immune responses to maintain homeostasis, and help prevent infections by pathogenic microorganisms. When the normal composition of the intestinal microorganisms is altered in *dysbiosis*, non-invasive bacteria can be transported to intestinal lymphoid tissue, leading to aberrant immune responses against microorganisms not normally considered a threat.

Macrophages and dendritic cells are the primary cells involved in maintaining tissue integrity and in initiating and controlling immune responses. These cells perform critical functions in preserving homeostasis and preventing infections. Macrophages and dendritic cells act to maintain tolerance to dietary antigens and control commensal and pathogenic microorganisms in the intestinal mucosa. They are distributed in lymphoid tissue such as Peyer's patches and are abundant in the lamina propria.

Dendritic cells are specialized antigen-presenting cells. These migratory cells participate in antigen trafficking and immunosurveillance. The intestinal network of these cells continually surveys the local microenvironment and assists in maintaining a balance between immune tolerance to harmless antigens and launching immune responses against intestinal pathogens. Dendritic cell stimulation leads to interleukin-12 secretion and a Th1 response, or interleukin-10 secretion and a Th2 response. Overall, dendritic cells act as sentinels that respond to inflammatory signals, capture luminal antigens, and migrate to intestinal lymphoid tissues to display such antigens to T cells. Their motility and plasticity allow dendritic cells to migrate from the lamina propria to the epithelium and the intestinal lymphoid tissue.

The cells of the lamina propria are critical in establishing bacterial tolerance and in orienting T cell immune responses. The effects of the intestinal microbiota on macrophages and dendritic cells appear to be essential for maintenance of intestinal immune homeostasis. Macrophages residing in the lamina propria learn to acquire non-inflammatory characteristics. Research has demonstrated that macrophages isolated from various regions of the intestine have differing modes of immune response indicating that distinct commensal microorganism populations in different regions of the intestine provide specific signals to macrophages and influence their immune profiles.

Th17 cells are a subset of CD4+ T cells and primarily secrete interleukin-17. They play a prominent role in intestinal mucosal host defenses as well as in development of autoimmune diseases. Components of the intestinal microbiota such as *Lactobacillus acidophilus* and *Bacteroides distasonis* stimulate Th17 cells in the intestine. Differentiation of Th17 cells is also triggered by cytokines, so Th17 cells can act as both protectors and aggressors, depending on environmental conditions. Their development is stimulated by commensal microorganisms, and can induce secretion of proinflammatory and anti-inflammatory cytokines. The intestinal microbiota and Th17 cells function in a regulatory feedback loop, and Th17 cells are important for maintaining equilibrium between the host and the microbiota.

As an example, *Escherichia coli Nissle* 1917 increased expression of zonula occludens and claudin proteins. *Bifidobacterium infantis Y1* secretes metabolites that cause increased expression of tight junction proteins. Administration of *L. plantarum* can enhance stability of tight junction complexes and mitigate their disruption by pathogens and inflammatory cytokines. Various probiotic microorganisms appear to regulate modifications in host cell signaling and as a result, tight junction protein complexes are stabilized and epithelial barrier function is promoted. Probiotics are capable of modulating epithelial barrier permeability, altering the inflammatory potential of epithelial cells, and directly regulating the activity of immune cells. By improving barrier function, probiotics and commensal microorganisms can reverse inflammatory reactions in intestinal epithelial cells caused by cytokines such as TNF-α. Different strains of probiotics have the ability to regulate activation of specific dendritic cells, directing subsequent T cell activity toward Th1, Th2, and Th17 responses. These probiotics include *Lactobacillus acidophilus*, *L. reuteri*, *L. rhamnosus*, and *Bifidobacterium bifidum*. Additionally, a synergistic effect between probiotics and immunoglobulin A (IgA) has been demonstrated.

Probiotics can reverse immunological disturbances by stimulating regulatory responses that mediate the balance between proinflammatory and anti-inflammatory cytokines. Stimulation of the immune system with probiotics can facilitate production of interleukin-10, an essential cytokine in the maintenance of intestinal homeostasis. The immunoregulatory effect of *Lactobacillus* leads to a reduction in levels of proinflammatory cytokines such as interleukin-6 and TNF-α. Research has demonstrated that *Lactobacillus* and *Bifidobacterium* activate dendritic cells.

Probiotics can also promote increased production and secretion of IgA by modulating expression of cytokines in the intestine. Additionally, they function as antagonists to pathogenic bacteria by triggering effects such as production of antibacterial molecules, reduction of intestinal luminal pH, and inhibition of bacterial adherence to the intestinal epithelium. *E. coli Nissle 1917* was the first probiotic reported to have beneficial effects in patients with inflammatory bowel disease.

Live probiotic bacteria can compete with pathogenic bacteria for nutrients, inhibiting growth and adhesion of such pathogens. Metabolites secreted by probiotics can strengthen tight junctions through cell signaling pathways. Promotion of tight junction integrity prevents pathogenic bacteria from translocating to the lamina propria through the paracellular pathway and initiating proinflammatory responses.

Research shows that the intestinal microbiota of diabetic and obese individuals differs from that of the healthy, non-obese population. Alterations in the intestinal epithelial barrier and the intestinal microbiota are implicated in the pathophysiology of diabetes, cardiovascular disease, and obesity. The constellation of these three disorders is termed *metabolic syndrome*. With such alterations and barrier disruption, bacteria and bacterial endotoxins are translocated from the intestine to the liver and other tissues, leading to low-grade chronic inflammation. Such translocations beyond the intestinal epithelial barrier are considered an important mechanism in the development of the chronic inflammation characteristic of metabolic diseases.

Disorders of Pregnancy, Infertility, and Osteoporosis Associated with Gluten Intolerance and Celiac Disease

Alison Harding recalled that as a teenager her menstrual cycle was always irregular. In 1996 at age 20, the hair on her head began to fall out. She had abnormal facial hair, acne, and had developed insulin resistance. At age 21, she was diagnosed with polycystic ovary syndrome (PCOS), a disorder in which enlarged ovaries contain multiple small fluid collections (cysts). Additionally, she had always been thin while living at her parents' home and eating traditional Vietnamese food. At 5 feet 7 inches tall, she weighed approximately 115 pounds, but when she went away to college and started eating breads and pasta, foods to which she was not accustomed, she gained an excessive amount of weight.

After graduation, she obtained full-time employment, was eating less, working out more, and was still more than 40 pounds overweight. She developed amenorrhea, an abnormal absence of menstruation, and consulted with an obstetrician specializing in infertility who prescribed metformin, an antidiabetic medication which helped reduce her PCOS symptoms. Her facial hair became less pronounced, she lost weight, and the number and size of her ovarian cysts diminished, but Alison was still not ovulating.

In her early 30s, Alison sustained a severe neck injury and began taking substantial quantities of ibuprofen. She gained another 40 pounds in less than three months and weighed 170 pounds. A friend told her about an article describing the relationship between gluten and infertility that referenced research demonstrating that 90% of women with PCOS were also gluten intolerant.

After investigating further, Alison started a gluten-free diet in 2010 at the age of 34 and lost 18 pounds in two weeks. Doctors had informed her that she had a short luteal phase and even if she conceived, the embryo wouldn't implant in her uterus. She had also been told that the chances of a woman with PCOS becoming pregnant are similar to those of a 45-year-old woman (typically estimated at 3–4%). Based on the professional advice they received, Alison and her husband were prepared to adopt until she became pregnant only six weeks after going gluten-free.

Her obstetrician advised her to remain on her gluten-free diet. She went off metformin during her first trimester, consulted with a specialist regarding gluten intolerance and celiac disease, and added specific foods to her diet so she could obtain sufficient carbohydrates and protein. Her pregnancy was uneventful and she successfully delivered a baby girl (now 4 years old). Alison also eliminated casein and peanuts from her diet as well as all antibiotics. With these new constraints in place, she lost an additional 26 pounds in one month. She continued treatment in our clinic, was not on any medications, and ovulated regularly for the first time in her life.

Regarding her gluten-free diet, Alison said that if she ingests gluten inadvertently, "I can feel my uterus contract as if I'm having labor pains," but overall, "I feel like I'm back to my early 20s." Her PCOS-related symptoms are "much better" and she can maintain a healthy weight of 135 – 140 pounds. She also maintains appropriate insulin levels with calorie restriction and regular cardiovascular exercise. She is thriving as a working mother and successfully managing her prior health conditions with a gluten-free diet and a few additional dietary controls.

Gluten Intolerance, Celiac Disease, Obstetrical Outcomes, and Infertility

Over the years, there has been an increasing awareness of the manifestations of gluten intolerance and celiac disease beyond the gastrointestinal tract, including such conditions as disorders of pregnancy, infertility, and osteoporosis. Infertility is defined as the impossibility of conceiving after 12 months of unprotected intercourse. It is relatively frequent, occurring in approximately 8–12% of couples that include a woman of childbearing age. An association between celiac disease and abnormalities of reproduction was first noted in a 1970 report that described three patients with untreated celiac disease and infertility. All three became pregnant after initiating a gluten-free diet.

Disorders of Pregnancy

With respect to outcomes of pregnancy, maternal celiac disease can influence fetal development in several ways. Gluten fragments such as gliadin induce cytokine production by monocytes and lymphocytes in the mother's bloodstream, which can negatively affect the fetus. Inflammation of the maternal intestinal mucosa causes suboptimal nutritional intake, leading to intrauterine growth retardation. Undiagnosed (and therefore untreated) celiac disease in a pregnant woman implies a metabolically active disorder, with attendant deleterious consequences for the fetus. Research demonstrates that women with celiac disease that was undiagnosed at the time of delivery were more likely to have a preterm birth, caesarean section, or offspring with low birth weight.

One study showed that women with celiac disease that was diagnosed during pregnancy gave birth to infants with a mean birth weight of 2,800 grams compared with 3,220 grams among women with no celiac disease. The increased risk of intrauterine growth retardation and low birth weight is related to insufficient nutrition. Research shows that pregnant women with undiagnosed celiac disease had lower placental weight than women with no celiac disease. Additionally, intrauterine growth retardation and low birth weight can be associated with maternal inflammatory processes and dysregulation of the maternal immune system caused by celiac disease.

Other studies have demonstrated that celiac disease is associated with high rates of unexplained infertility, spontaneous abortion, and stillbirth. Women with celiac disease have a shortened reproductive period with delayed menarche (the first menstrual cycle), amenorrhea, and early menopause. These clinical entities may be the initial findings that ultimately lead to a diagnosis of celiac disease. With respect to obstetrical outcomes, latent celiac disease (assessed on the basis of tissue transglutaminase antibody titers) was more than seven times as likely to be present in a group of women whose pregnancies were associated with intrauterine growth retardation, five times as likely in a group with recurrent spontaneous abortion, more than four times as likely in a group with stillbirth, and more than four times as likely in a group with unexplained infertility. One study showed the relative risk of spontaneous abortion is 8.9 times higher in pregnant women with untreated celiac disease.

In a study done in Italy, published in 2000, 845 pregnant women were screened for celiac disease. Twelve newly diagnosed cases were identified. In these twelve there had previously been seven unfavorable outcomes of pregnancy. Three infants had died and one was born prematurely. One woman had pre-eclampsia (high blood pressure in pregnancy), and one had a breech delivery. Five of the women with celiac disease delivered small-for-gestational-age infants and three additional infants were delivered prematurely. Five women had been pregnant more than once. Four of these five had experienced at least one miscarriage.

The mean age of diagnosis of celiac disease is increasing and being diagnosed more commonly in women who do not have classic symptoms of malabsorption (such as diarrhea, abdominal bloating, gas, and weight loss). This silent presentation of celiac disease combined with delayed diagnosis results in prolonged exposure to gluten and greater injurious effects on a woman's reproductive capacity and fertile life span. It is well known that celiac disease increases the risk of recurrent miscarriages, premature delivery, low birth weight, and early menopause. These complications diminish once a gluten-free diet is instituted.

Regarding pathophysiology, research has demonstrated that placentas in pregnant women with celiac disease appear to be abnormal. It has been proposed that maternal antibodies generated in celiac disease negatively impact placental health and function. For example, placental tissue transglutaminase may be bound by maternal anti-tissue transglutaminase antibody, with resultant compromise to placental activities. Research suggests that placental tissue transglutaminase is important in stabilizing dying cells, ensuring their clearance by phagocytic cells and preventing inflammatory reactions. Additionally, tissue transglutaminase may have a role in the organization and structure of the syncytiotrophoblast microvillous membrane that acts as an interface between the placenta and maternal blood. Tissue transglutaminase expression and cell death are reported to be increased in trophoblast cells, suggesting injury to both the fetal and maternal portions of the placenta. Further, decreased availability of tissue transglutaminase, owing to binding by maternal anti-tissue transglutaminase antibody, may lead to defective interactions between the placenta and the maternal circulation with adverse effects on fetal health such as intrauterine growth retardation, premature birth, and low birth weight.

A women's health survey in 2015 evaluated 970 women, including 641 with no history of celiac disease and 329 with biopsy-proven celiac disease. A significantly higher prevalence of spontaneous abortions was identified in the celiac disease population compared to the control group. Additionally, women with celiac disease had a higher prevalence of preterm delivery compared to controls. Another study demonstrated that delivery of a preterm infant is linked to subsequent assessment of underlying celiac disease in the mother. Parents of 905 preterm infants were screened for celiac disease using anti-endomysial antibodies and anti-tissue transglutaminase antibodies. A higher prevalence of celiac disease in mothers of low-birth-weight infants was found.

A 1999 study conducted in Denmark examined 211 babies born to 127 mothers with celiac disease and compared these newborns to 1,260 control deliveries. Low birth weight (less than 2,500 grams—5 pounds 8 ounces) occurred in 12.3% of babies born to mothers with celiac disease. Following treatment for celiac disease, consisting of a strict gluten-free diet, subsequent birth weights were comparable to those in the control women.

Another study demonstrated that women with undiagnosed celiac disease have an 8.9 relative risk of abortion and a 5.8 relative risk of delivering a low-birth-weight infant. Relative risk compares the probability of an event occurring in an exposed group to the probability of the event occurring in a non-exposed group.

Infertility

Gluten intolerance and celiac disease are also risk factors for infertility. These disorders are also known to delay menarche (a young woman's first menstrual cycle) and cause early menopause. The overall effect is the shortening of a woman's reproductive cycle by several years.

Infertility may be the first symptom of celiac disease. A 1996 study in Finland evaluated 98 women who were seen at a university hospital for infertility. Up to the time of their hospital examination, there was no known cause for infertility in any of these patients. Four women (4.1%) were found to have celiac disease, a frequency many times higher than that for celiac disease in the general population at 1%. Overall, between 4 to 8% of women with unexplained infertility have celiac disease. Numerous case reports have demonstrated successful resolution of infertility after diagnosis of celiac disease and treatment with a gluten-free diet.

A recent meta-analysis evaluating 4,471 subjects demonstrated a significant association between women with a diagnosis of infertility and celiac disease with an odds ratio of 3.09. An odds ratio indicates the likelihood that an outcome will occur given a particular exposure, compared to the likelihood of the outcome occurring in the absence of that exposure and it is a relative measure of effect. The study concluded that undiagnosed and untreated celiac disease is a risk factor significantly associated with infertility in women.

Screening of women for gluten intolerance and celiac disease may be of great value in cases involving reproductive disorders, infertility, and complications of pregnancy. The question regarding which groups to screen was addressed in a 2009 article. Couples experiencing infertility of unknown cause and women in specific risk groups will benefit from screening for celiac disease. Women with autoimmune diseases, a family history of gluten intolerance or celiac disease (for example, an affected first-degree relative), and/or a history of anemia are at a higher risk for celiac disease and represent populations for whom screening is critically important.

All physicians need a high index of suspicion for gluten intolerance and celiac disease. In pregnant women, celiac disease can be suggested by persistent iron deficiency anemia as well as abnormal weight loss during the first two trimesters. Both conditions are related to malabsorption. It is important to recall that celiac disease can demonstrate no symptoms or show symptoms unrelated to the gastrointestinal tract. Screening of pregnant women, particularly those with a family history of gluten intolerance and celiac disease is an important preventive measure.

Treatment dramatically reduces the rate of obstetric complications in pregnant women with celiac disease. Up to 50% of women with untreated gluten intolerance and celiac disease experience a miscarriage or other unfavorable outcome of pregnancy. With proper treatment, a strict gluten-free diet, the occurrence of such obstetric problems reduces to the level found in the general population.

Celiac Disease, Gluten Intolerance, and Bone Disease

Many studies have demonstrated reduced bone mineral density in adults with untreated celiac disease. Such persons may present with bone pain, muscle weakness, and pathological fractures. A meta-analysis reported in 2008 demonstrated a 43% increased risk of fracture in patients with celiac disease. With respect to bone disorders, patients with celiac disease often have osteopenia, osteoporosis, or osteomalacia.

Osteopenia is loss of bone density (reduced bone mass), which can be caused by normal aging or a variety of conditions including malabsorption syndrome, diabetes, and cancer. Research demonstrates that celiac disease patients had significantly lower bone mineral density at the lumbar spine and top of the femur (femoral neck) than control subjects. Up to 41% of newly diagnosed celiac disease patients had low bone mineral density for age (greater than one standard deviation below normal) at the lumbar spine and 39–50% had low bone mineral density for age at the femoral neck. There is an increased prevalence of fracture in celiac disease patients owing to loss of bone mineral density. A meta-analysis reported in 2008 evaluated a total of more than 20,000 celiac disease patients and more than 96,000 controls. The study described a 43% greater risk of fracture in those with celiac disease.

Osteopenia in celiac disease is rapidly reversible. In one study, after one year of a gluten-free diet the percentage of patients with severe osteopenia in the spine decreased from 9 to 5% and in the femur from 14 to 9%. (Severe osteopenia is defined as greater than two standard deviations below normal bone mineral density.) Studies have demonstrated normal bone mineral density in patients with celiac disease who have adhered to a strict gluten-free diet for more than four years.

Osteoporosis involves loss of bone tissue and disorganization of bone structure. It is bone loss specifically associated with metabolic factors that primarily affects weight-bearing bones including the pelvis, femur (thigh bone), and lumbar vertebra. Such bone loss can result in disabling fractures.

Osteomalacia refers to inadequate or delayed mineralization of the bone matrix in adult bone, resulting in softening of bones. A similar process in children is termed rickets and involves interruption in the orderly development and mineralization of the growth plates of long bones. Both osteomalacia and rickets are related to deficiencies in vitamin D metabolism.

Osteoporosis is usually painful, the pain being caused by microfractures within the bone tissue. Fractures of the entire bone can also occur, typically in the hip and lumbar vertebras. A wrist fracture is likely if a person with osteoporosis falls on an outstretched arm. Patients with undiagnosed and untreated celiac disease have an increased risk of fractures, suggesting possible osteoporosis. A study conducted in Argentina, published in 2000 found that 25% of 165 patients with celiac disease had experienced one or more fractures, compared to 8% in 165 hospital controls.

Osteoporosis in celiac disease results from persistent inflammation of the intestinal epithelial mucosa, atrophy of intestinal villi, and alterations in intestinal absorption (malabsorption). In malabsorption, the ability of the small intestine to absorb calcium, amino acids (the building blocks of protein), and vitamin D is greatly compromised. Each of these ingredients is essential for the formation of strong bones. Over time the deficit of raw materials causes a decrease in bone mass.

Lowered serum levels of calcium induce a compensatory increase in serum levels of parathyroid hormone which leads to an increase in bone resorption (bone destruction). When resorption of bone is faster than new bone formation it results in a net loss of bone and osteoporosis. Additionally, local and systemic inflammation has a role in the pathology of bone loss in celiac disease. Chronic inflammation is characterized by an increase in proinflammatory cytokines in the intestinal mucosa and bloodstream, including tissue necrosis factor-α (TNF-α), interleukin-1, and interleukin-6. These cytokines stimulate the growth and differentiation of osteoclast cells that resorb bone tissue. In untreated celiac disease patients, higher serum cytokine titers are correlated with loss of bone mineral density.

In severe cases of classic celiac disease, malabsorption causes reduction in serum calcium and vitamin D levels. These deficits lead to secondary hyperparathryroidism with resultant increased bone remodeling, reduced bone mass, alteration of bone quality, reduced bone strength, and increased risk of fracture. Research shows that more than 75% of adult patients with untreated celiac disease and an overt malabsorption syndrome at the time of diagnosis have loss of bone mass. Loss of bone mass affects approximately 50% of patients with subclinical celiac disease who have minimal, transient, and seemingly unrelated symptoms.

Osteoporosis can occur in children who have gluten intolerance and celiac disease, but with a gluten free diet, osteoporosis in children usually resolves completely. In adults, loss of bone mass and osteoporosis are also alleviated by following a gluten-free diet. Eliminating all sources of gluten reduces chronic inflammation in the person's small intestine, and nutrients begin to be absorbed normally. Normal bone mass begins to be restored and symptoms and risk of fracture reduce and resolve.

In one study, patients with celiac disease were followed for up to five years while on a gluten-free diet. Bone mineral density increased or remained stable in 52% of patients at the lumbar spine and in 68% at the femoral neck. These findings show that bone disorders in patients with celiac disease may recover during long-term adherence to a gluten-free diet. Following a strict gluten-free diet for one year results in significant improvement (5–8%) in bone mineral density. Following it for two years improved bone mass and improved levels of serum markers of bone and mineral metabolism. In children, normalization of bone mineral density levels can be reached in as early as two years following initiation of a strict gluten-free diet. Persistent bone loss compared to the normal population in celiac disease patients maintaining a gluten free diet can be related to chronic inflammation. Thus, early detection of celiac disease leads to improved outcomes.

Laboratory Testing for Atypical Cases of Celiac Disease

Screening studies evaluating serum antibody titers have shown that up to 1–2% of the Western population may be affected by celiac disease, but owing to the varying clinical presentation of celiac disease, the condition remains markedly undetected. Research has identified anti-endomysial IgA (immunoglobulin A) antibodies and antibodies to tTG as sensitive serological markers of celiac disease. tTG is the most widely distributed member of the transglutaminase family. These laboratory tests should be utilized to evaluate the presence of celiac disease in patients with unexplained infertility, disorders of pregnancy, or bone disease.

Anti-endomysial antibodies are directed against the endomysium, the outer connective tissue membrane that surrounds smooth muscle bundles that contain a form of tissue transglutaminase. Chronic inflammatory responses associated with gluten intolerance and celiac disease disrupt and cause destruction of the intestinal epithelial lining. Disruption of the endomysium in intestinal mucosal smooth muscle causes endomysial tissue transglutaminase to be recognized by the immune system as non-self with subsequent production of antibodies against this enzyme (anti-endomysial antibodies). Anti-endomysial antibodies are present in patients with celiac disease and in those with dermatitis herpetiformis, a skin disorder present in up to 4% of patients with celiac disease. Research has demonstrated that the concentration of anti-endomysial antibody titers correlates with the severity of abnormalities in the intestinal mucosa.

Tissue transglutaminase is localized to the lamina propria, the highly vascular layer of connective tissue underlying the intestinal epithelial cells. It has many functions, including actions related to the creation of the intercellular matrix, the gel-like substance that holds cells together. In the small intestine, tissue transglutaminase interacts with gluten protein fragments, causing deamidation that primes gluten fragments to be recognized as non-self and capable of launching a widespread immune response. When tissue transglutaminase changes a gluten fragment in the process of deamidation, the modified gluten protein structure causes it to be recognized and taken up by HLA DQ2 and DQ8 antigen-displaying proteins. In a series of responses, the body now reacts to the gluten proteins as a threat.

Owing to its high specificity, anti-endomysial antibody serology is considered the gold standard in laboratory evaluation of potential celiac disease. Patients with celiac disease may not present with classical gastrointestinal symptoms such as abdominal bloating, pain, gas, diarrhea, and weight loss. There may be a wide variety of extraintestinal symptoms including joint pain, arthritis, osteoporosis, infertility, and neuropsychiatric complaints. An elevated anti-endomysial antibody titer is an excellent predictor of celiac disease in those with subtle, minimal, or atypical symptoms.

The National Institutes of Health Consensus Panel Statement on celiac disease recommends serological testing as the first step in demonstrating the presence of celiac disease. Anti-endomysial antibodies and anti-tissue transglutaminase antibodies are the primary serological tests utilized in such evaluations. Anti-endomysial antibodies are correlated with intestinal epithelial mucosal pathology, with more severe intestinal atrophy corresponding with higher antibody titers. Research has shown that anti-endomysial antibodies have a diagnostic sensitivity of 93% and a specificity of 100%. Sensitivity is the ability of a diagnostic test to detect the condition being evaluated when the condition is, in fact, present. Specificity is a measure of how often a positive diagnostic test accurately predicts the presence of the condition being evaluated.

Another study investigating the diagnostic effectiveness of anti-endomysial antibodies and anti-tissue transglutaminase antibodies demonstrated sensitivities of 93% for both and specificities of greater than 99% and 98%, respectively, in the diagnosis of celiac disease with atrophy of intestinal villi. A review of studies comparing endomysial antibody with human recombinant tissue transglutaminase antibody shows that endomysial antibody more often has a higher specificity. Human recombinant tissue transglutaminase antibody more often has a higher sensitivity.

Celiac disease is often associated with serious disorders that affect physiological systems remote from the gastrointestinal tract, including infertility, disorders of pregnancy, and bone disease. Celiac disease may present with such atypical findings. An accurate diagnosis depends on the clinical acumen and expertise of the patient's physician. With a high index of suspicion, such a physician can order serum antibody titers and place the patient on a gluten-free diet. Excellent outcomes can be obtained with strict adherence to a gluten free diet, including a much anticipated and hoped-for pregnancy and successful delivery of a healthy baby in the case of celiac disease–associated infertility, and improved bone mass and bone health in the case of celiac disease associated bone disorders.

Probiotics and Prebiotics

Awareness and Mindfulness

Robbie Mendoza was an all-American teenager with more than a few natural gifts. Not only was he a member of his high school jazz band, he was also the drum major for his school's marching band, which was an authentic triple threat: a skilled musician, an accomplished performer, and an inspiring leader. As drum major, Robbie led the marching band's rehearsals, taught the drill charts, and conducted the field shows. Additionally he was a member of the National Honor Society who participated in the two-year International Baccalaureate Diploma Program. As part of his International Baccalaureate Diploma community service, Robbie volunteered at Habitat for Humanity, an organization that builds affordable housing for low-income families in the United States and around the world.

At the age of 15, Robbie experienced a significant health problem while participating in humanitarian service in Ensenada, Mexico, where he was helping provide basic necessities to impoverished people in the local communities. The mission was Robbie's first trip to Mexico and he said he, "ate a lot of flour", which is a primary ingredient in tortillas, a staple of the Mexican diet.

Robbie soon felt sick after every meal, becoming nauseated with severe, stabbing abdominal pains and diarrhea. He completed his two-week mission and upon his return to San Diego, his parents brought him to our clinic, thinking that his problems were caused by drinking the water in Ensenada. Which was one of our concerns as well, so we ordered the necessary tests. Robbie's blood tests showed an iron deficiency, antibodies to gluten, and autoantibodies associated with celiac disease. His symptoms weren't a result of drinking contaminated water, they came from gluten intolerance. We started him on a gluten free diet, multivitamins, and iron supplements. "I began to feel much better right away," Robbie said.

Since then, he has become more knowledgeable about his family medical history. "Both my Mom and my grandmother have celiac disease," he said. "We've been gluten-free in my house for years, but, you know, you don't think you're going to have any problems. I mean, I've always been real healthy." He smiled at a memory. "You hate to hear the doctor say you're gluten intolerant, because you know what it means. No more pizza when you go out with friends. No more spaghetti dinners when you're over at their house, but that's the price you pay. I don't want to be sick. It doesn't feel good. Not at all."

After being on his gluten-free diet for almost four years, Robbie said, "I feel fine when I'm gluten free. That's why I stick to the diet." When asked what his advice might be for teenagers with similar medical issues, he said, "Pay attention to what's going on. Don't delay. That's important. If you feel bad, go see the doctor. Doing community service taught me about awareness and mindfulness. Kids usually don't think about these things too much, but awareness and mindfulness actually have a lot to do with good health and staying healthy."

The Human Gastrointestinal Tract

The human gastrointestinal tract is host to approximately 100 trillion bacteria. These microorganisms have evolved to obtain the energy they need to survive from their human host and in exchange they help support the physiological, metabolic, and immune system capabilities that have contributed to our evolutionary success. More than 1,000 individual microbial species have been identified in the human gastrointestinal (GI) tract. The collective genome of the human intestinal microbiome encodes approximately 3 million genes, more than 100 times the 30,000 genes encoded by human DNA. The large intestine contains the majority of GI microbes, as many as 100 billion microorganisms per milliliter of fluid in the GI lumen.

Numerous studies have demonstrated that these commensal microorganisms (the habitual residents of the gut) engage in extensive interactions with their host's GI function, metabolism, and immune system. The composition and activity of the microbiome markedly influences human health and disease.

The intestinal microbiome interacts with the immune system to maintain homeostasis in healthy states and promote inflammation in states of dysbiosis, in which the composition of the microbial community becomes imbalanced. Dysbiosis has been observed in many diseases including: celiac disease, inflammatory bowel disease, obesity, type 1 diabetes, rheumatoid arthritis, and other autoimmune conditions. It frequently results in chronic inflammatory and autoimmune processes, not only within the GI tract, but also in remote sites including the skin, brain, muscles, and joints.

Dysbiosis and Celiac Disease

It is well established that persons affected by poorly controlled celiac disease have demonstrable dysbiosis. Compared to healthy individuals, people with active celiac disease have higher numbers of Gram-negative intestinal bacteria (such as *Escherichia coli* and *Pseudomonas aeruginosa*) known to activate proinflammatory processes and lower numbers of Gram-positive intestinal bacteria (such as *Lactobacillus* and *Bifidobacterium*) that are associated with anti-inflammatory responses. Research demonstrates that quantities of potentially pathogenic microorganisms such as *Staphylococcus*, *Salmonella*, *Shigella*, *Klebsiella*, and *Bacteroides* are significantly higher in children with celiac disease than in healthy children. Studies of children with celiac disease demonstrate that even strict compliance with a gluten-free diet does not completely restore the normal intestinal microbiota. Supplementation of a gluten-free diet with probiotics and prebiotics helps ameliorate dysbiosis and is an important addition to the maintenance protocol of patients with celiac disease.

The adult microbiota is relatively stable, but its composition is influenced by diet, use of medication, disease, and aging. GI tract microbes can be commensal or transient, and may be beneficial, harmful, or pathogenic. Beneficial microbes such as *Bifidobacterium* and *Lactobacillus*, usually ferment carbohydrates and do not produce toxins. They engage in crosstalk with the host immune system. Such interactions between the microbiota, immune cells, and the intestinal epithelium affect immune system homeostasis and metabolic activities in the GI tract. Additionally, commensal microorganisms inhibit pathogens by competing for nutrients and stimulate the immune system. They also promote digestion and absorption of nutrients, synthesize vitamins and proteins, inhibit the growth of potential pathogens, and reduce cholesterol. The intestinal microbiome substantially increases the host's ability to obtain nutrients from food. This increased digestive capacity supplements the limited diversity of complex carbohydrate metabolizing enzymes that are encoded in human genes. As a result, intestinal microorganisms limit the resources available to intestinal pathogens. Homeostasis of the intestinal microbiome directly influences our health and well-being.

Microorganisms in the first part of the large intestine meet their energy requirements by fermenting carbohydrates and dietary fiber that have escaped digestion in the small intestine. Foods rich in dietary fiber include fruit, vegetables, legumes, and grains. Carbohydrate sources contained in dietary fiber include oligosaccharides such as fructo-oligosaccharides and galacto-oligosaccharides, other sugars such as lactulose and non-absorbed lactose, and mannitol. Fermentation by *Bifidobacterium*, *Lactobacillus*, and *Bacteroides* produces short-chain fatty acids (SCFA), acetic acid (acetate), propionic acid (propionate), and butyric acid (butyrate). All SCFA contribute toward the host's daily energy requirements.

SCFA are absorbed into the bloodstream, transported to the liver, muscles, and peripheral tissues, and are used as an energy source, contributing 7–8% of the host's daily energy requirements. Acetate is metabolized in the brain and muscles. Propionate is metabolized in the liver and used to generate ATP (*adenosine triphosphate*), a primary energy source utilized in many physiological functions. Propionic acid can reduce production of cholesterol by the liver. Butyric acid promotes normal differentiation and proliferation of large intestine epithelial cells. Butyrate is a major energy source for the epithelial cells lining the large intestine and may have anti-cancer properties.

SCFAs have been shown to directly inhibit activity of important gastrointestinal pathogens and act to lower pH in the large intestine which inhibits growth of potential pathogens and promotes growth of beneficial bacteria such as lactobacilli and bifidobacteria. SCFAs also help regulate sodium and calcium absorption. In animal models, the addition of SCFAs in intravenous feeding increased helper T cells, neutrophils, and macrophages, and increased the activity of natural killer (NK) cells. Overall, the addition of probiotics to the diet helps restore balance to the intestinal microbiome by altering the intestinal pH, producing antimicrobial substances such as SCFAs and bacteriocins, thereby competing with pathogenic bacteria for nutrients. Probiotic activity also helps repair the intestinal epithelial barrier.

Gastrointestinal Structure and the Immune System

Research consistently demonstrates that colonization of the GI tract by a sufficiently diverse microbiome is critical for proper development and regulation of innate (inborn) immunity and adaptive (learned) immunity. Deviation from a healthful composition of intestinal microorganisms leads to loss of immune and metabolic homeostasis.

The GI tract can be considered the body's largest immune organ. Its lining represents the body's greatest area of mucosal contact with the environment and contains approximately 80% of all antibody-producing cells. Antigens deriving from the intestinal microbiome as well as from microorganisms in the environment are critical for development and maturation of gut-associated lymhpoid tissue (GALT) and modulation of the immune response.

These immune system cells constantly survey the contents of the intestinal lumen to detect undesirable antigens and protect the intestinal epithelial mucosa against harmful pathogens while modulating inflammatory responses to various antigens, and scavenging dead cells. Specialized epithelial cells such as M cells are located immediately above Peyer's patches and engulf antigens from the intestinal lumen. The antigen is then delivered to intraepithelial lymphocytes and macrophages which migrate to lymph nodes in the lamina propria where an immune response may be initiated.

Paneth cells, located at the bases of intestinal epithelial villi are arrayed with numerous pattern recognition receptors (PRRs) and are specialized for production and release of specific antimicrobial molecules, including defensins which are triggered by interactions between Paneth cell PRRs and microbe-associated molecular patterns (MAMPs) displayed on the surface of intestinal pathogens. MAMPs are generally invariant structural components of bacteria. The lock-and-key action of a specific MAMP with its associated PRR stimulates an individualized immune system response and cytokine release, leading to either tolerance or a proinflammatory cascade. Sensing of MAMPs stimulates growth and development of intestinal epithelial cells and arms them for release of antimicrobial molecules, if needed. These host regulatory events have broadly protective effects, but increased stimulation results in cellular inflammation and cell death.

Dendritic cells sample and capture antigens in the lumen by extending cytoplasmic branches between adjacent intestinal epithelial cells. They sense microbes through PRRs and migrate to lymphoid patches containing naive T cells. Dendritic cells behave as antigen-presenting cells by presenting foreign antigens to T cells, potentially initiating an adaptive immune response. Dendritic cells also transport commensal bacteria to mesenteric lymph nodes, where commensal-specific immunoglobulin A (IgA) antibody responses are generated. Secretion of these specific immunoglobulins and their transport into the lumen enables tolerance of commensal microorganisms. Overall, the body's predominant IgA production occurs in the immune tissues of the GI tract. IgA antibodies bind to microorganisms and pathogen-derived toxins, neutralizing these cells and proteins, preventing access to host intestinal epithelial cells.

What are Probiotics and Prebiotics?

In the early 1900s, Elie Metchnikoff, the Nobel Prize–winning scientist, observed longevity in Bulgarian peasants and associated this with their elevated consumption of sour milk. He hypothesized that GI tract function could be enhanced by introducing exogenous, food-borne bacteria into the gut. Such *probiotic* ("for life") bacteria have been defined by the Food and Agriculture Organization of the United Nations as "live microorganisms which when administered in adequate amounts confer a health benefit on the host", (FAO/WHO, 2006), but not every live microorganism contained in a food is a probiotic. Probiotics must be able to exert benefit to the human body through growth and/or activity, but they are transient.

Some may be able to persist and replicate in the GI tract for a few days, but disappear soon after cessation of their intake. A probiotic microorganism must be able to survive in the GI tract until it reaches that portion of the tract where it will exert its intended effects. Probiotics must be able to compete successfully with microorganisms resident in the GI tract. Overall, generation of probiotic metabolites results in the production of immunoregulatory signals that suppress intestinal mucosal immune reactions and enhance nutrition.

The concept of prebiotics developed more recently. The term prebiotic was invented in the mid-1990s. Prebiotics are defined as "a selectively fermented ingredient that results in specific changes in the composition and/or activity of the gastrointestinal microbiota, thus conferring benefit(s) upon host health" (Gibson et al, 2010). The prebiotic concept is based on the premise that the intestinal tract already contains beneficial microorganisms. A prebiotic is a nondigestible food ingredient that benefits the host by targeting specific components and altering the composition of the GI microbiome. Its primary targets are intestinal lactobacilli and bifidobacteria, with a primary focus on bifidobacteria.

Prebiotics, that is, dietary carbohydrates, increase the metabolic capacity of selected commensal bacteria. The prebiotic is material that is selectively fermented, stimulating the growth and activity of specific microorganisms, shifting the intestinal microbiome toward a more advantageous composition. Prebiotics preferentially stimulate microbial gene expression that affects regulation of immune function. Many of them share the regulatory definition of dietary fiber, but prebiotics are differentiated by the selectivity of their fermentation. The main prebiotic site of action is the large intestine, one of the most diversely colonized and metabolically active organs in the human body.

Prebiotics are comprised of non-digestible oligosaccharides, carbohydrates that consist of three to nine saccharide units. Many occur naturally in foods such as asparagus, Jerusalem artichokes, leeks, garlic, onions, and oats, however the overall intake of prebiotics in the typical Western diet is small. An effective approach is to fortify more frequently consumed foods with prebiotic ingredients which can be added to bread, yogurt, ice cream, and drinks. The target level for prebiotic intake is from 2 to 20g per day. These amounts can be easily incorporated into foods like yogurt, cereals, and drinks. Prebiotics as well as probiotics must be consumed regularly to demonstrate a consistent benefit.

Bifidobacterium and *Lactobacillus* in the large intestine preferentially ferment undigested carbohydrates (prebiotics), resulting in a reduced luminal pH. A lower pH in the large intestine supports the growth and survival of commensal microorganisms that prefer acidic conditions and inhibits the ability of some pathogens to adhere to the intestinal epithelial lining and translocate across the epithelial barrier or colonize the GI tract. Fermentation of prebiotics by *Bifidobacterium* yields acetic acid and lactic acid. Metabolism of these products by other microbial species yields butyric acid and propionic acid. Butyrate and propionate are also produced by the direct fermentation of other undigested carbohydrates. Butyric acid enhances mucosal cell differentiation and promotes the integrity of the intestinal epithelial barrier.

Additionally, research demonstrates that prebiotic administration is followed by production of bacteriocins by commensal microorganisms. Bacteriocins are protein toxins that inhibit the growth and survival of competing pathogenic bacteria.

Probiotic Activities and Immune System Function

Commensal microorganisms in the GI tract have the ability to protect the host from pathogens and modulate activity of the host immune system. Dysbiosis perturbs immune regulatory networks that normally inhibit intestinal inflammation and contributes to proinflammatory responses directed toward antigens of commensal microorganisms, contributing to gastrointestinal disease, such as celiac disease, inflammatory bowel disease, and systemic autoimmune disease, such as rheumatoid arthritis, type 1 diabetes, and multiple sclerosis. It is also linked to obesity and metabolic syndrome. Administration of probiotics, primarily *Lactobacillus* and *Bifidobacterium*, acts to normalize the composition of intestinal microorganisms and restore immune system homeostasis. As an example, *L. reuteri* and *B. bifidum* activity inhibits interleukin-12 release and may be of importance in reestablishing immune system balance in Th-1 mediated diseases.

Probiotics support and enhance intestinal epithelial barrier function. Their administration leads to increased production of mucin proteins and increased development of the mucous layer that protects intestinal epithelial cells from translocation of pathogenic microorganisms. Both probiotics and prebiotics enhance the structure of intestinal epithelial tight junctions by increasing expression of genes coding for occludin and claudin protein families.

Probiotics which are ingested bacteria such as *Bifidobacterium* and *Lactobacillus* and prebiotics which stimulate specific commensal microorganisms interact with gastrointestinal lymphoid tissue and immune system cells to modulate the immune and inflammatory responses of the host. Different strains of probiotics are able to regulate dendritic cell activation, polarizing subsequent T cell activity toward Th1 (*L. acidophilus*), Th2 (*B. bifidum*), and Th17 (*L. rhamnosus* GG). Research indicates that a Th1-mediated response is predominant in celiac disease and a Th2-mediated response is predominant in ulcerative colitis. Th17 cells, which produce interleukin-17, are crucial for control of chronic inflammatory disease such as multiple sclerosis and Crohn's syndrome.

Administration of probiotics such as *L. rhamnosus* GG (a strong inducer of transforming growth factor-beta [TGF-β] and interleukin-1β) could affect development and maturation of Th17 cells and ameliorate clinical symptoms of chronic inflammatory disease. *L. rhamnosus* GG produces signaling molecules that help prevent intestinal epithelial cell death that otherwise would have been induced by proinflammatory cytokines. Laboratory models of colitis indicate that one of these protein signaling molecules is active in protecting intestinal epithelial cells from injury and inflammation.

Promotion of cell survival when proinflammatory cytokines have been released by activated immune cells represents an important probiotic effect contributing to homeostasis. Such effects are enhanced by addition of probiotics to the diet. Overall, *Lactobacillus* species induce growth and development of regulatory T cells, upregulate interleukin-10 and TGF-β, and increase local IgA production by B lymphocytes in the lamina propria.

This modulation of immune and inflammatory responses also impacts tissues and organs beyond the GI tract. Toll-like receptors (TLRs), located on intestinal epithelial cells like dendritic cells and M cells mediate the interaction between intestinal microbes and host cells. TLRs are a class of pattern recognition receptors. Their activation launches a specific signaling pathway leading to the expression of nuclear factor-κβ (NF-κβ), proteins that function as transcription factors that regulate expression of genes influencing innate and adaptive immunity, inflammation, and B-lymphocyte and other lymphoid tissue development. Regarding inflammation, NF-κβ expression leads to the production of a large range of cytokines including TNF-α and interleukins. Probiotics such as *Bacteroides* and *Lactobacillus* inhibit activation of the classical NF-κβ pathway and downregulate proinflammatory gene expression.

Additionally, activation of TLRs initiates a cascade of immune signals and differentiated maturation of helper T cells (Th1, Th2, and Th17) and regulatory T cells, providing an appropriate response to specific pathogens. Th1 cells promote cell-mediated immune responses involving phagocytic cells such as macrophages and neutrophils. Th2 cells promote humoral immunity and are involved in antibody production. Th1 cells fight viruses and other intracellular pathogens and help to eliminate cancerous cells. Th2 cells act to combat extracellular organisms.

Th17 cells are thought to be the most ancient of helper T cell subsets and may have evolved to strengthen intestinal epithelial barrier defenses to promote tolerance of the intestinal microbiota. Th17 cells have a pivotal impact in immune homeostasis and inflammation, producing multiple cytokines and influencing a wide range of intestinal cell targets. The Th17 pathway has a prominent role in development of adaptive immunity to intestinal microorganisms. Also, the Th17 pathway has a propensity for provoking an inflammatory response promoted by interleukin-17 and interferon-γ. This pathway is now understood as a major contributor to the pathogenesis of inflammatory bowel disease and autoimmune disease.

Many genes associated with innate and adaptive immunity pathways are integrated with the Th17 response with involvement in maintaining intestinal epithelial barrier integrity and repair, microbial sensing, and secretion of immunomodulatory cytokines. Intestinal microorganisms are a potential environmental factor in the development and persistence of autoimmune disease, so the constitution of the intestinal microbiota, that is commensal microorganism homeostasis versus dysbiosis, is increasingly implicated in maintenance of health versus development of inflammatory and autoimmune diseases.

Regulatory T cells counterbalance proinflammatory factors by stimulating expression of interleukin-10 and other anti-inflammatory cytokines. In a healthy intestinal environment, T cells act together with B lymphocytes, dendritic cells, phagocytes, and intestinal epithelial cells to prevent commensal microorganisms from causing damage to the host.

Toll-like receptor activation also results in B cell differentiation and secretion of IgA into the intestinal lumen. Research demonstrates that the interaction between commensal bacteria and TLRs located on dendritic cells and other immune system cells located in the intestinal epithelium is necessary for intestinal homeostasis and prevention of intestinal injury. If these interactions are deregulated by dysbiosis, tissue damage and chronic inflammation can occur. Inflammatory bowel disease and autoimmune disorders including celiac disease and type 1 diabetes are associated with a pathological immune response to intestinal microorganisms. Regular consumption of probiotics helps repair damaged intestinal epithelial tissues and reduce symptoms of these diseases by restoring intestinal microbial balance and contributing to immune system homeostasis.

Additionally, probiotics and prebiotics stimulate increased production of anti-inflammatory cytokines such as interleukin-10 and TGF-β and decreased expression of proinflammatory cytokines such as tissue necrosis factor-alpha (TNF-α) and interferon-gamma (IFN-γ). Such effects likely represent mechanisms by which probiotics and prebiotics mitigate chronic intestinal inflammation. Probiotics and prebiotics also impact the innate immunity response through modulation of the activity of NK cells and phagocytic cells (neutrophils and macrophages).

Microbiome host signaling is reciprocal and involves the immune system, the nerve system within the GI tract, and host metabolic systems. Microorganism signaling is required for immune system development and homeostasis. Conversely, a functional immune system is necessary for maintenance of a healthy microbiome. A depleted microbiome may result in immune system deficits. Defects in immune system function can lead to altered composition in the GI microbiome. Interactions between the immune system and intestinal microorganisms are critical in maintaining homeostasis across the intestinal epithelial barrier and in protecting against infections occurring at mucosal sites and inflammatory diseases involving the intestinal mucosa.

Key questions focus on the definition of a commensal microorganism and how the host distinguishes between beneficial and harmless commensals and dangerous opportunistic pathogens. The distinction between commensal and pathogenic microorganisms is not always clear. As molecular patterns involved in recognition of pathogens are also expressed by commensal, nonpathogenic microorganisms, detection of such patterns is only part of the process. The response decision, that is the determination by the immune system as to whether a specific microorganism is friend or foe is based partly on signals from intestinal microorganisms such as expression of the immunomodulatory polysaccharide, polysaccharide A, produced by *Bacteroides fragilis*.

Polysaccharide A signals through regulatory T cells and suppresses Th17 effector cells, avoiding an inflammatory immune response and promoting colonization of the host's GI tract by *B. fragilis*. The host employs a cell-to-cell surveillance system allowing it to respond to danger and maintain equilibrium within the composition of the intestinal microbiome. Research demonstrates that even a single intestinal bacterial species can be sufficient to shift homeostatic balance in the direction of tolerance or inflammation. *B. fragilis* is an example of a commensal microorganism that supports anti-inflammatory responses by activating regulatory T cells with subsequent production of interleukin-10. The induction of Th17 cells by commensal segmented filamentous bacteria (SFB) provides protection against intestinal pathogens, but in alternate circumstances, as in dysbiosis, SFB can induce differentiation and activation of Th17 cells with subsequent production of the proinflammatory cytokine interleukin-17. Th17 cells retain a capacity for divergent function and cytokine expression.

In dysbiosis, changes in the intestinal environment provoke an increase in segments of the microbiome that cause disease and/or a decrease in commensal microorganisms that exert a beneficial effect on the host. Dysbiosis creates an imbalance in immune system responses by innate and adaptive immunity resulting in an inflammatory cascade with subsequent compromise of the intestinal epithelial barrier, disruption and destruction of intestinal epithelial cells, and clinical disease. A single commensal bacteria species can prompt a local immune response, which can trigger development of an autoimmune disease at remote sites such as the bones and joints (as in rheumatoid arthritis) or the central nervous system (as in multiple sclerosis).

Patients with rheumatoid arthritis have defective regulatory T cell function with increased numbers of Th17 cells and increased levels of interleukin-17 in the serum and synovial tissue (the membrane lying between the ligamentous joint capsule and the joint cavity of synovial joints). Such alterations in immune system function represent a break in immune tolerance to commensal microorganisms, prompted by dysbiosis followed by a proinflammatory response that can lead to local intestinal epithelial pathology and autoimmune tissue damage and disease at remote sites.

Probiotics strengthen and repair tight junctions and enhance intestinal epithelial barrier function, modulate activities of commensal microorganisms and their interactions with the host, competitively exclude pathogens, and modulate immune cell activity and cytokine profiles. Immunomodulatory properties of probiotics involve various cell types, signals, and receptors. Distinct classes of probiotics express distinct microbe-associated molecular patterns (MAMPs) recognized by specific pattern recognition receptors (PRRs) located on dendritic cells. Toll-like receptos and other PRR signaling elicited by probiotic MAMPs contribute to small intestine defense systems, preventing bacterial penetration of host tissues. Probiotic stimulation of regulatory T cells contributes to the production of TGF-β and interleukin-10, which are critical mediators of immune homeostasis. TGF-β is a primary inducer of development of IgA-producing B lymphocytes. The main role of IgA antibodies is to establish tolerance with commensal microorganisms.

Comparative genomic analyses of probiotic bacteria have identified a set of approximately 125 genes that are suggested to contribute to intestinal epithelial mucosal and systemic immune responses. Numerous protein markers displayed on the cell surface of probiotic microbes interact directly with host intestinal epithelial cells and immunomodulatory cells.

Use of Probiotics and Prebiotics: Modulation of the GI

Microbiome

Adding live microorganisms to the diet is a well-known method for modulating the composition of the intestinal microbiome. Early records show that humans have been consuming bacterial drinks for more than 2,000 years. In the early 1900s, the zoologist Elie Metchnikoff hypothesized that certain intestinal microorganisms adversely affect the host and consumption of other bacteria could reverse such effects. Working at the Pasteur Institute in Paris, Metchnikoff refined his treatment method by using pure cultures of Lactobacillus, which is used to ferment milk to produce traditional yogurt. Later, researchers leveraged Metchnikoff's work as the basis for studies on what became known as probiotics which contain large numbers of living cells capable of surviving and exerting metabolic activity in the GI tract, and providing benefit to the host.

Probiotics exert a beneficial impact on dysbiosis including control of yeast (*Candida albicans*) overgrowth. Probiotics facilitate elimination of pathogenic bacteria such as *Clostridium difficile* and *Helicobacter pylori*, reduce local and systemic inflammatory responses, prevent autoimmune and allergic reactions, and act to lower serum levels of cholesterol. Further, probiotics reduce concentrations of cancer-promoting enzymes and metabolites in the GI tract. Laboratory studies demonstrate that *Bifidobacterium lactis*, a live probiotic, inhibits the toxic effects induced by wheat gliadin (a large protein fragment derived from partial digestion of gluten) in intestinal epithelial cells. Mouse models show that probiotics prevent intestinal damage in celiac disease.

Clinical experience demonstrates that appropriately selected probiotics significantly reduce bloating and diarrhea in patients with gluten intolerance and celiac disease. Their use reduces gluten-associated joint and muscle pain, fatigue, brain fog, and decreases yeast colonization of the GI tract. Administration of probiotics normalizes markers of inflammation such as C-reactive protein and markers of intestinal mucosal immune responses such as secretory immunoglobulin A. Typically, probiotic administration requires at least 4-6 months to demonstrate measurable results.

Choosing appropriate probiotic strains may be challenging for the inexperienced consumer. Probiotic bacteria that may benefit persons with celiac disease and gluten intolerance include the following:

- *B. lactis*
- *Bacillus coagulans (also known as L. sporogenes)*
- *Bifidobacterium bifidus*
- *L. casei*
- *L. plantarum*
- *L. rhamnosus*
- *L. salivarius*
- *Lactobacillus acidophilus*
- *Lactococcus lactis*
- *Saccharomyces boulardii*

L. acidophilus DDS-1 is one of the best characterized probiotic strains worldwide and occurs naturally in the human GI tract and many dairy products. Its administration results in the production of B vitamins, vitamin K, and lactic acid, which help maintain beneficial microorganisms in the GI tract. It also helps prevent colon cancer and inhibits development of gastric/duodenal ulcers caused by *H. pylori* and it acts to reduce serum cholesterol levels, reduce symptoms of lactose intolerance, and reduce intestinal pain.

L. plantarum is found in fermented foods such as sauerkraut, pickles, kimchi, and some cheeses. Its administration results in production of lactic acid and hydrogen peroxide, which kills pathogenic bacteria. It also acts to synthesize the amino acid L-lysine, which promotes absorption of calcium and growth of muscle tissue. Additionally, *L. plantarum* is of benefit for persons with pancreatic insufficiency.

Administration of *L. casei*, found in yogurt, cheddar cheese, fermented green olives, and *L. rhamnosus*, found in yogurt, cheese, and fermented milk results in production of lactic acid in the large intestine, which kills pathogenic bacteria.

Pediococcus is isolated from kimchi, a traditional Korean food consisting primarily of fermented cabbage. It acts to normalize the intestinal microbiome and assists in healing yeast infections.

B. bifidus, found in buttermilk, kefir, kimchi, and sauerkraut administer results in modulation of intestinal immune responses; production of vitamin B, vitamin K, and folic acid; and production of hydrogen peroxide. Its activities also assist in preventing colon cancer.

Research suggests that B. *lactis*, found in enriched yogurt and milk, directly modulates the function of intestinal epithelial cells. It increases expression of a hormone-like pathway critical for maintenance of intestinal epithelial integrity and downregulates expression of proinflammatory enzymes. Overall, it can inhibit intestinal epithelial damage caused by gluten/gliadin and is potentially beneficial for people with celiac disease and those with gluten intolerance. Intake of B. *lactis* can accelerate intestinal epithelial recovery after initiating a gluten-free diet and can provide protection against traces of gluten in the environment and in some supposedly gluten-free products.

Lactococcus lactis is used in the production of cheese and buttermilk. Administration of L. *lactis* results in production of lactic acid, which helps maintain beneficial microorganisms in the GI tract, and fermentation of lactose, which reduces symptoms of lactose intolerance.

Saccharomyces boulardii microorganisms persist in the gastrointestinal lumen and act to restore and maintain commensal microorganisms. Research demonstrates the efficacy of S. *boulardii* in the treatment and prevention of numerous GI disorders. Potential indications for its use include irritable bowel syndrome, ulcerative colitis, Crohn's disease, partial IgA deficiency, peptic ulcer disease owing to H. *pylori*, infection with C. *difficile*, and diarrhea (traveler's diarrhea and antibiotic-associated diarrhea).

B. *coagulans* (L. *sporogenes*) is characterized by increased survival in the acidic gastric environment and the bile acid associated duodenal environment. It is activated in the lower GI tract and releases anti-inflammatory molecules. Additionally, it helps eradicate intestinal microorganisms responsible for inflammatory immune responses. Activated B. *coagulans* produces bacteriocins and lowers local pH by producing lactic acid, helping eliminate pathogenic microorganisms that may be contributing to an inflammatory response. B. *coagulans* also produces SCFAs such as butyrate, an energy source for epithelial cells lining the large intestine and a modulator of the intestinal epithelial immune system.

To achieve therapeutic responses, the daily dose of probiotics should be at least 25 billion colony-forming units (CFUs) and should be taken with plenty of water on an empty stomach either 20-30 minutes before breakfast or 1-2 hours after dinner. Taking probioitcs on an empty stomach is preferred because when we eat, stomach acid is produced which kills the beneficial microorganisms found in probiotics. For persons taking antibiotics, the timing of probiotic administration must be separated from antibiotics administration by at least several hours.

Summary

Gluten intolerance and celiac disease are associated with aberrant microorganisms in the entire gastrointestinal tract, including the oral cavity. Such altered composition of the intestinal microbiome can contribute to specific abnormalities in immune system function observed in patients with celiac disease. These abnormalities, including low production of secretory immunoglobulin A, and decreased levels of natural killer cells, predispose development and perpetuation of autoimmune diseases. A gluten-free diet alone is not the ultimate solution to ameliorating dysbiosis and normalizing the intestinal microbiome. The continuous life-long use of probiotics and prebiotics in conjuction with a gluten-free diet is highly recommended to help repair and restore the structure and function of the gastrointestinal tract and reestablish immune system homeostasis.

The Way Forward

Stan Woodson, recently retired, worked with computers all his life. Stan laughingly calls himself a "dinosaur," stating that he used to work with computers that "filled up an entire room and needed full-time air-conditioning or they would go on the fritz. In those days computers were big, clunky machines. There were no MacBooks, no Windows, no color displays. None of that. You ran programs by inserting a deck of punch cards. That's right. Cardboard punch cards with a bit of computer code punched into each of them. That's how old I am."

Stan spent some years in the military before embarking on a long career as a systems analyst for the Department of Energy. Stan recalls, "But when I started getting close to the time I'd planned on retiring, my body just kind of fell apart. It was the darnedest thing."

In 2011, Stan began having persistent pain in his jaw. Friends said there might be a problem with his heart, so Stan went to see his family doctor, but nothing seemed to be wrong and his doctor prescribed pain relievers. Stan took the prescription, but didn't fill it, thinking he could handle the pain. It didn't get worse, but it didn't go away either, and after a few more weeks Stan noticed swelling on both sides of his face near the back of his jaw, then his fingers became swollen and painful. "They hurt so much," Stan said. "I couldn't even wring out a washrag." Soon his toes also became swollen and painful, and he had difficulty walking, so Stan called his doctor who recommended he consult with our clinic.

Stan told us about his recent problems and the periodic diarrhea he had suffered for many years. Lab tests identified elevated autoantibodies characteristic of gluten intolerance, celiac disease, and additional autoimmune disorders. Stan was placed on a three month trial of a gluten and dairy free diet. He lost 25 pounds, going from 175 to 150 pounds, all his pain subsided, the swelling around his jaw went away, and his fingers and toes returned to normal.

Stan also learned that his swollen fingers and toes were caused by lupus (which can lead to a variety of symptoms) and the pain and swelling around his jaw were caused by Sjögren's syndrome. Both conditions are autoimmune disorders related to or caused by the body's immune reaction to gluten. We also placed Stan on Plaquenil as part of his treatment for lupus.

"Altogether it took one or two years to be feeling pretty good," he said. "By then the pain and swelling were all gone and the diarrhea was a lot less frequent." Previously, he felt sick, feverish, and his skin itched all the time. After being on a gluten free diet and taking Plaquenil for four years, Stan has improved dramatically. "I feel very good 90% of the time. I need to see my optometrist every so often because of possible side effects of Plaquenil, but they're not common and I'm not worried. I'm in very good shape thanks to Dr. Shikhman and a gluten free diet."

Regarding lifestyle changes and what it takes to be sure his diet is gluten free, Stan said, "I'm very careful with my special diet. Like most people, I used to eat out a lot. Being on a gluten free diet means you're eating at home much more, and my wife is very supportive. She helps me with whatever I need. The diet does take work, of course. You don't just roll out of bed and become gluten free. Like when I go out for an entire day, I need to pack a lot of my own food. Sometimes I hesitate to do things because of a lack of access to food, but then I remind myself that all I need to do is make a little extra effort and everything works out fine."

Treatment for Gluten Intolerance and Celiac Disease

As discussed, the origins of gluten intolerance and celiac disease are similarly complex, involving genetic and environmental factors. In addition to ongoing exposure to gluten, environmental triggers can include acute viral and bacterial infections of the gastrointestinal tract. Given these complex interactions and such a wide variety of symptoms, effective management of gluten intolerance and celiac disease involves multiple strategies and multiple modes of treatment.

Diagnosis of Gluten Intolerance and Celiac Disease

The first outcome for a patient in any medical interaction is to receive an accurate diagnosis. This is often not a straightforward process in gluten intolerance and celiac disease. In many cases the correct diagnosis can elude a patient for years. Sometimes the correct diagnosis is only obtained by accident, a result of severe symptoms that bring the person to the attention of a well-informed rheumatologist or gastroenterologist. Even in the 21st Century many physicians remain unaware of these conditions, and gluten intolerance and celiac disease are under-diagnosed to a significant extent.

Part of the challenge is that gluten intolerance and celiac disease are great mimickers. If a physician has an appropriately high index of suspicion, a young patient with chronic diarrhea or constipation, abdominal pain and/or abdominal bloating, nausea or vomiting, and lower-than-average height/weight metrics should bring gluten intolerance and celiac disease to mind, but often none of these signs or symptoms is present. The patient may not have any classical signs and symptoms of celiac disease. In such situations, the physician's skill level and diagnostic ability become very important.

A person with gluten intolerance and celiac disease may predominantly show signs and symptoms of anemia and complain of weakness and fatigue, difficulty concentrating, irregular heartbeat, mood changes, and/or headache. If all of these are present, anemia is a likely diagnosis, but thyroid disease is also possible. Depression can also be responsible for these symptoms. Celiac disease is typically further down the list of likely suspects, and only a very good diagnostician would consider it.

In another example, a person can complain of weakness and fatigue, fever, and muscle and joint pains which sounds like influenza, but the pains and fever come and go, which is uncharacteristic of an infection. By the time symptoms have persisted for a month or more, most people want to see a doctor. This set of symptoms suggests various rheumatologic autoimmune disorders including lupus, rheumatoid arthritis, polymyositis, and scleroderma. Celiac disease can cause identical symptoms and needs to be considered whenever autoimmune problems are part of the differential diagnosis. A person can have both celiac disease and a second or even a third autoimmune disorder.

Pediatric disorders require careful evaluation. In one case, a six-year-old child cried every night. It's often difficult to understand why a child is crying, but the parents finally discovered that their daughter had pain in her lower back and legs. The parents were at a loss to explain it, but their pediatrician knew such symptoms could indicate a serious problem such as bone cancer. Tests were done that demonstrated loss of bone density, indicating that the child had osteoporosis. Juvenile osteoporosis is rare and may be caused by kidney disease, hyperthyroidism, or type 1 diabetes. It can also be caused by malabsorption syndrome, a disorder found in celiac disease. Again, it is the awareness of celiac disease and its various modes of expression that leads to accurate diagnosis.

Consider the case of infertility. A married couple is trying to start a family. After a year without success, they begin a process of trying to determine whether the potential father and mother are physiologically capable of bringing a baby into the world. Everything checks out. They're reminded that nature takes its own course, and their doctors encourage them to keep trying. One day while searching the Internet for information on infertility, the wife reads about a possible connection to celiac disease. She remembers that her aunt and a cousin had it, and calls her doctor to ask if any tests can be done. She's referred to a rheumatologist who orders a series of lab tests that show autoantibodies in her blood associated with celiac disease.

Gluten intolerance and celiac disease are frequently primary underlying causes of unsolved medical problems. Awareness of gluten intolerance and celiac disease provides a key to accurate and timely diagnosis as well as effective treatment.

Accurately diagnosing difficult cases is the hallmark of an outstanding physician. Such skill requires intelligence and a heightened sense of awareness, what we've referred to as an elevated index of suspicion. At leading medical schools around the country, attentive medical students are reminded that "you see what you look for and recognize what you know." Experienced physicians inform their students that it doesn't take any particular effort to consider the obvious. It's easy to recognize what you know, but when a patient's symptoms represent an unfamiliar combination, as they often do in cases of gluten intolerance and celiac disease, the situation requires innovative, outside-the-box thinking.

Cases that are considered difficult and interesting account for less than 10% of a typical physician's practice. The other 90% are fairly straightforward. No patient wants to be an unusual or interesting case, but gluten intolerance and celiac disease are interesting, and such cases can only be correctly understood by well-trained, well-informed, insightful physicians.

Patients with gluten intolerance and celiac disease would benefit greatly if these conditions became commonly recognized by a majority of doctors, pediatricians, and internists. Such patients would become much more typical, less "interesting," and receive accurate, timely diagnoses rather than being tested in error for other conditions and placed on numerous trial medications, referred to countless specialists, and experiencing numerous side effects while suffering ongoing symptoms.

Standard diagnostic procedures and treatment programs for gluten intolerance and celiac disease have existed for quite a while.

How to Diagnose Gluten Intolerance and Celiac Disease?

Celiac disease is a likely diagnosis if a child has several of these signs and symptoms:

- Abdominal bloating
- Abdominal pain
- Anemia
- Constipation
- Diarrhea
- Malnutrition
- Markedly short stature
- Markedly underweight
- Nausea
- Vomiting

For accurate diagnosis in teenagers and adults, it is essential to remember that gluten intolerance and celiac disease may show none of these findings. Instead, signs and symptoms typical of various other conditions are commonly present.

If gluten intolerance and celiac disease are suspected, blood tests are done to detect the presence of characteristic autoantibodies. The most accurate of these *serum immunoglobulin tests* measures levels of anti-tissue transglutaminase antibody (tTG). An increase in anti-tTG antibody concentration is found in almost all cases of celiac disease.

A second immunological test measures anti-gliadin antibodies which are less predictive of celiac disease as they are identified in other diseases as well, but anti-gliadin antibodies indicate the presence of gluten intolerance. When either test is positive, a three-month trial of a gluten free diet is recommended as a key component of treatment.

Testing for genetic markers can also be performed. More than than 97% of patients with celiac disease have HLA DQ2 and/or HLA DQ8 antigen-displaying proteins. A positive test indicating the presence of DQ2 and DQ8 genes is a very strong predictor that a person has gluten intolerance and celiac disease.

Additionally, the doctor may recommend a biopsy of the small intestine. Small tissue samples are obtained using an endoscope, a thin flexible tube. Biopsy material is evaluated for the presence of characteristic changes associated with the chronic inflammation of celiac disease, however a small intestinal biopsy is not particularly sensitive, as many people with gluten intolerance and celiac disease do not have such inflammatory changes. In other words, you can have celiac disease and have a normal-appearing small intestine.

The gold standard for diagnosis is the body's response to a three month gluten free diet. If the tTG autoantibody is present and/or the person tests positive for the HLA DQ2 or HLA DQ8 genetic marker, the next step is to begin a strict gluten free diet. If the patient's symptoms have improved by the end of the three-month trial, then gluten intolerance and/or celiac disease is an accurate diagnosis. It's important to remember that other diseases, including autoimmune diseases, can also be present. Regardless, a strict gluten-free diet is the first step on the road to recovery.

The Four-Step Treatment Program

Gluten intolerance and celiac disease cause inflammatory and immunological reactions that can affect numerous body systems. Any or all of the digestive, musculoskeletal, endocrine, reproductive, nervous, and cardiovascular systems can be involved in these disease processes. Effective treatment necessarily involves a comprehensive approach.

- Step One: a gluten-free diet for life.
- Step Two: restoring metabolic balance and treating hormonal imbalances.
- Step Three: normalizing the immune response and treating autoimmune diseases.
- Step Four: tumor monitoring and surveillance.

Step One—A Gluten-Free Diet for Life

Dietary gluten is the trigger and root cause of every symptom of gluten intolerance and celiac disease. In a genetically susceptible individual prolonged exposure to dietary gluten provokes an immunological reaction, which becomes chronic if the gluten exposure persists. As we've discussed, the prolonged immunological response causes an inflammatory reaction, and these two processes feed on each other. The combined immunological/inflammatory reaction then spreads to other organ systems, and a range of symptoms develop.

Treating symptoms like diarrhea, abdominal pain, fever, anemia, and fatigue is very important, but this treatment doesn't affect the underlying cause. The only action that helps prevent problems from worsening, provide symptomatic relief, and begin to heal the damage is a gluten free diet for life.

No one wants to be told they have gluten intolerance or celiac disease. The patient knows a substantial lifestyle change is about to begin, and none of us is ever eager for that and there's no way to cushion the blow. Truth and full disclosure are always the best policies. Caring doctors, in addition to being accurate diagnosticians, are supportive, provide all the necessary information, and emphasize the many benefits of living a gluten-free lifestyle.

A gluten free diet is the foundation and most essential element of treatment. All sources of gluten are identified, eliminated, and replaced if possible with gluten free substitutes. In the early weeks and months of the diet, hidden sources of gluten are revealed. The patient feels better, then they don't. They know they're doing a good job of being gluten free. They cleaned out their refrigerator and kitchen cabinets and thoroughly washed dishes, utensils, and cookware. Highly motivated to find the gluten containing or gluten retaining culprits, they read all the labels on all the food they have in the house. Aha! The bottle of Tuscan salad dressing they bought at the natural foods store contains malt vinegar. Something about it rings a bell and they call a friend who has celiac disease. "That's right," the friend says. "Malt is made from barley which contains gluten." Every day the patient learns more and becomes more skilled in ways that help them to be healthy and well.

Why is a strict gluten free diet necessary? First, gluten intolerance and celiac disease are *permanent* conditions. The patient is sensitized to gluten and even the slightest bit provokes an immune reaction. A concentration as low as 20 parts per million (0.002%) can cause symptoms in a gluten intolerant person. Some people's gluten intolerance has led to serious problems including autism, schizophrenia, Addison's disease, type 1 diabetes, rheumatoid arthritis, lupus, and infertility. Others have serious symptoms related to celiac disease itself, including severe abdominal pain, persistent diarrhea, constipation accompanied by intense pain, and/or signs and symptoms of malnutrition. None of these individuals wants to experience a return of symptoms and each has learned through experience that there's a direct relationship between symptoms and gluten. They know being gluten free takes work and they are willing to do it.

In the case of autoimmune diseases associated with gluten intolerance, a cascade effect exists between gluten intake, immunological response, and inflammatory reaction. Even a small amount of gluten can provoke a disproportionate inflammatory response. As the cellular and tissue destruction caused by lupus, Addison's disease, or Graves' disease can be cumulative and permanent, avoidance of gluten is the best policy.

Occasionally the temptation to take a bite of a friend's slice of pizza or to have a slice of double fudge chocolate layer cake becomes too great. Some people are passionate about cheese Danish and others crave a croissant with their morning coffee, so a person might fall off the gluten free wagon for a brief indulgence. Usually uncomfortable symptoms ensue and the person must weigh whether the negative outcome is worth the momentary enjoyment.

Fortunately, a person on a gluten-free diet is no longer doomed to a life of deprivation. As we'll learn in the next chapter, a wide variety of high quality gluten free foods are available. Gluten free ingredients, foods, and products have become an important niche market and the selection is continually expanding. A substantial gluten free industry has developed, commanding display and shelf space in markets and bookstores as well as page views and purchasing power on the Internet.

People on gluten free diets have an abundance of choices and a wide opportunity for culinary pleasure and delight. Do you crave chocolate chip cookies? There are plenty of delicious gluten-free recipes available. What about blueberry crumble, banana cranberry muffins, or cherry vanilla ice cream? With a little time and energy, all of these delectable foods can become part of a regular gluten-free diet.

Pizza. "Rye" bread, Coffee cake, Challah, all of these foods can remain integral parts of a regular menu. Once a person learns where to find them or how to make them, they've added considerably to their quality of life. Being on a gluten free diet does not require deprivation. Gluten free substitutes are available for almost all familiar gluten containing foods, and there's always the interesting alternative of learning how to cook the foods that the patient and their family wish to have.

For someone on a gluten free diet for life it's important not only to be gluten free, but to ensure their diet is nutritionally complete. Many people who are gluten intolerant or have celiac disease will be recovering from a greater or lesser degree of malnutrition. For these people, complete nutrition is especially critical. For others who did not have digestive tract symptoms, complete nutrition remains a priority.

When a person begins a gluten-free diet it may feel as if they've eliminated everything they used to eat, which is a reasonable perception. Gluten is not only a staple of the Western diet, it is also used as filler and stabilizer for many prepared and packaged foods. As a result, people on gluten free diets have often wondered exactly how they were going to obtain the nutrition they need.

The primary concern is sufficient protein. The U.S. RDA is 0.8 grams of protein per kilogram body weight which is a minimum requirement. For a 120-pound woman that's approximately 45 grams of protein per day. A 180-pound man needs about 68 grams of protein per day. Again, these quantities are the barest minimums. More protein is always better, particularly if you're exercising regularly.

For people regularly doing moderate exercise, a more accurate calculation of daily protein requirement uses a ratio of 0.75 gram of protein per pound of lean body mass. You can easily obtain an approximate measure by using one of the many lean body mass calculators available on the Internet. For a man who is 6 feet tall and in good shape, weighing 180 pounds, lean body mass is approximately 145 pounds, so he needs approximately 110 grams of protein per day. For a woman who is 5 feet 3 inches tall and in good shape, weighing 120 pounds, lean body mass is approximately 94 pounds. She needs approximately 70 grams of protein per day.

Four ounces of salmon fillet contains about 25 grams of high-quality protein, as does four ounces of ground lean sirloin. Four ounces of fresh boneless-and-skinless chicken breast contains about 24 grams of high quality protein and four ounces of fresh turkey breast contains about 20 grams of high quality protein. Basically, four ounces of fish, poultry, or beef provides approximately 24 grams of protein.

Fresh eggs contain the highest quality complete protein available, in fact egg protein is used as the reference standard against which all other protein sources are compared. A whole egg contains approximately 6 grams of protein. Dairy products are next highest in terms of overall quality. For lacto-ovo vegetarians, eggs, milk, yogurt, and gluten free cheese are excellent protein sources. An 8-ounce glass of milk contains approximately 8 grams of protein, and a cup of yogurt contains approximately 12.

Vegetarians need to be sure they're getting a complete protein every day that contains all the essential amino acids. Combining certain foods ensures you're getting what you need. A combination of beans and gluten-free bread provides complete protein, as does a corn-and-beans dish. Additional complete protein combinations include nut butter and gluten free bread. Rice and beans, lentils, or peas also provide complete protein. Eating seeds, nuts, and a variety of vegetables is another means of obtaining complete protein during the course of the day.

In addition to obtaining sufficient protein, people on a gluten free diet need to eat plenty of fresh fruits and vegetables. These colorful foods provide a wide range of vitamins, minerals, and phytonutrients, small biochemicals required for good health. Phytonutrients are powerful antioxidants that help prevent cellular damage, reduce inflammation, and help minimize the effects of chronic disease. You can't get phytonutrients in a bottle. They are designed to work together in combinations that can only be obtained by consuming the foods themselves. Eating a variety of colorful fresh fruits and vegetables ensures you're getting the range of phytonutrients needed to help overcome the effects of gluten intolerance and celiac disease.

Drinking sufficient water every day is another key element of a gluten free diet. Eight glasses of water a day is a good average. Four glasses per day is a good place to start if you haven't been drinking much water in a while. Start with four glasses and build up to eight per day.

Drinking water has two main purposes. First, water hydrates our cells and tissues. Our bodies are composed of approximately 70% water, so we need sufficient water to maintain that percentage and stay healthy. Water is the environment in which all our cellular functions take place. Drinking enough helps our cellular mechanisms and processes run properly. Not enough means things are going to go wrong, which implies eventual sickness and disease. Water also helps remove the toxins and other chemical end products that build up from normal physiological activities like digesting food and building new cells. In this way, drinking pure water flushes out our systems. Other fluids such as tea and juice already contain dissolved materials, so they don't function as cleansers and purifiers. Drinking pure water is a key to good health.

Many people who begin a gluten free diet discover they're eating much healthier than they were previously. Being on a diet that's critical to their health requires them to engage in the food choices they make. We all know that our levels of health are directly related to the quality of food we eat, but knowing something doesn't always translate into taking effective action. There's no intrinsic motivation, but when our doctor says that to stop being sick we need to be on a gluten free diet for life, that's highly motivating and when a doctor specifies all the things we need to be doing, like eating gluten-free foods, high quality protein, and fresh fruits and vegetables, as well as drinking plenty of water, we're going to make sure we start developing these new habits.

The medical results of a gluten free diet are usually anticipated by one's doctor, but the personal results are often not anticipated by the patient. People on gluten-free diets discover they have more energy, get more restful sleep, and their ability to concentrate and do meaningful work is increased. They get more done during the day than ever before. They *want* to exercise and have more fun. They also become inspirations not only to themselves, but to their families and friends. In many cases, a person's entire perspective on life changes as a direct result of being on a gluten free diet that makes them healthy for the first time in years.

Step Two: Restoring Metabolic Balance and Treating Hormonal Imbalances

As we've seen, people with gluten intolerance and celiac disease can have a number of metabolic disorders, diagnosed and undiagnosed, as a result of malabsorption. The degree of malabsorption varies depending on the extent of gastrointestinal inflammation. Vitamins and minerals are poorly absorbed in malabsorption syndrome and various deficiencies can ensue. Additionally, different patients are susceptible to different metabolic imbalances.

Osteoporosis can result from calcium and vitamin D malabsorption. Iron deficiency anemia and vitamin B12 deficiency anemia can also result from malabsorption. Vitamin B deficiencies can result in irregular heartbeat, high blood pressure, weakness and pain in the legs, mood swings, and depression. Vitamin A deficiency can result in night blindness, corneal inflammation, and dry skin, while vitamin E deficiency can cause pain, numbness, and tingling in the extremities, as well as problems with muscular coordination and balance. Vitamin K deficiency can cause clotting disorders.

Any of these deficiency diseases can be related to gluten intolerance and celiac disease. Metabolic balance can be restored by vitamin and mineral supplementation once a gluten-free diet has been in place for at least 30 days.

Osteoporosis is treated with high doses of vitamin D and calcium supplementation. Vitamin D should be obtained as vitamin D3, the naturally occurring and active form of the vitamin. As a supplement, calcium is absorbed more effectively in the form of calcium lactate. For iron deficiency anemia, iron supplements should be in the form of iron-chelate (iron bound to an amino acid), which facilitates absorption. Vitamin B12 supplementation is best obtained with sublingual tablets. By allowing the lozenge to dissolve under the tongue, vitamin B12 is absorbed directly into the bloodstream, bypassing slower and less efficient absorption through the digestive tract.

Iron, calcium, vitamin D3, and vitamin B12 deficiencies are addressed with high-dose supplements. Additional minerals and vitamins, such as A, E, and B complex can be obtained through high-dose multivitamin tablets or capsules. These products contain well-balanced combinations of vitamins, minerals, and trace elements needed to address deficiencies and restore metabolic function.

It is important to insure that your vitamin/mineral supplements are gluten free. It's possible for gluten to be an ingredient in the manufacturing process of pills, tablets, and capsules. Your supplements should be free of gluten and other common allergens, and contain no artificial flavors, colors, or preservatives. If necessary, check with the manufacturer to be certain.

Hormone Imbalances

Hormone imbalances are related to the overall metabolic landscape of gluten intolerance and celiac disease. Two such imbalances, elevated prolactin levels (hyperprolactinemia), and elevated parathyroid hormone levels (secondary hyperparathyroidism) can be associated with celiac disease.

Prolactin stimulates the mammary glands to enlarge during pregnancy and stimulates them to produce milk after childbirth. Research has discovered an additional role of prolactin in modulating the immune response. Prolactin is produced by many cells including nerve cells and immune system lymphocytes. It is elevated in celiac disease and many autoimmune diseases such as lupus, rheumatoid arthritis, type 1 diabetes, and Addison's disease. The immune cascade in celiac disease causes elevated prolactin levels, which cause an even greater immune response.

A gluten free diet helps reduce the immunological and inflammatory reactions of gluten intolerance and celiac disease, indirectly leading to reduction in prolactin levels. Addressing the hormonal imbalance of elevated serum prolactin may also require medications such as cabergoline and bromocriptine.

Increased parathyroid hormone levels are caused by vitamin D deficiency and/or calcium deficiency. Elevated parathyroid hormone causes calcium to be withdrawn from bone, resulting in bone pain, swollen joints, and possible fractures. A gluten free diet treats the malabsorption caused by gluten intolerance and celiac disease, restoring normal absorption of vitamin D and calcium. Additionally, high-doses of vitamin D3 and calcium may be needed to treat secondary hyperparathyroidism and restore parathyroid hormone levels to normal.

Step Three: Normalizing the Immune Response and Treating Autoimmune Diseases

In many cases of gluten intolerance and celiac disease, chronic inflammation of the inner lining of the small intestine leads to structural changes. The convoluted surface of this inner lining (which under a microscope looks like a mountain range) becomes flattened. This flattening is known as *villous atrophy*. Atrophy of the villi (microscopic fingerlike projections of intestinal tissue) results in malabsorption.

Gluten intolerance and celiac disease can alter the composition of bacteria that normally inhabit the small intestinal tract, known as microflora. When a person is healthy, microflora assists in the process of digestion. These microorganisms help prevent growth of harmful species, help train the immune system, and even synthesize vitamins like biotin and vitamin K. Colonies of normal microflora are destroyed by ongoing inflammation, and harmful species are able to take hold and multiply. The presence of harmful bacteria causes an immune response against them, resulting in a continual cycle of immunological and inflammatory reactions.

An important component of treatment of gluten intolerance and celiac disease involves restoring normal intestinal microflora. Reestablishing these healthful bacteria helps break the cycle of chronic immune response and inflammatory reaction. Colonies of healthful bacteria are restored by consuming specific foods and supplements known as *probiotics* and *prebiotics*.

Probiotics are living microorganisms that are safe for human consumption and provide many physiological benefits. They promote the growth of "good" intestinal microflora, suppress the growth of "bad" bacteria, help regulate the immune response, and help strengthen the intestinal barrier. Prebiotics are indigestible carbohydrates that increase the population of certain intestinal bacteria. After consumption, prebiotics reach the colon where they are fermented by anaerobic bacteria. Short-chain fatty acids are produced, as well as carbon dioxide and hydrogen gas. The acid balance in the colon increases favoring the growth of "good" bacteria that is normal intestinal microflora.

An additional component of step three activities is the medical treatment of autoimmune disorders, if present. Various pharmaceuticals may be needed to counter the effects of lupus, rheumatoid arthritis, autoimmune thyroiditis, Sjögren's syndrome, scleroderma, polymyositis, polyarteritis, and Addison's disease. Such medications may include Prednisone or prednisolone, hydrocortisone, methotrexate, Neoral, Zyrtec, or Plaquenil. A rheumatologist will be able to provide appropriate recommendations, advice, guidance, and follow-up.

Step Four: Tumor Monitoring and Surveillance

Inflammatory diseases and infections can lead to malignant changes in the affected tissues. It does not occur frequently, but is more common in certain disorders including celiac disease. For example, colon cancer is ten times more common in those with gluten intolerance and celiac disease than in the general population. Additionally, individuals with celiac disease are at increased risk for the following:

- Adenocarcinoma of the small intestine
- Carcinoma of the mouth and throat
- Esophageal carcinoma
- Lymphoma
- Melanoma

A 2003 study demonstrated that 43 (11%) of 383 patients with celiac disease also had a diagnosis of cancer. Nine individuals had non-Hodgkin's lymphoma (only one case was expected based on prevalence in the general population). Five had melanoma (one case expected). Three had adenocarcinoma of the small intestine (0.1 case expected) and three had esophageal carcinoma (0.3 case expected). These findings represent a range of increased risk from five to 30 fold, depending on the type and location of malignancy. For non-Hodgkin's lymphoma, other studies have reported a range of increased risk from three to 100 fold.

Monitoring for possible development of malignancy in patients with gluten intolerance and celiac disease is a critical and possibly life-saving step in their long-term management. Periodic blood tests should be done to measure specific biochemicals that indicate the presence of a malignant change. Additionally, periodic examinations and tests should be done to detect the possible presence of tumors.

The good news is that many studies have shown the benefits of a gluten free diet in reducing the risk of cancer. Periodic monitoring and maintaining a gluten free diet for life helps reduce cancer risk and helps keep people healthy and well.

For people with gluten intolerance and celiac disease, the way forward is clear. The four key steps must be followed to reduce symptoms, remain relatively symptom free, and achieve optimum health and well-being. Some actions are done daily, others once a year or less. Regardless, new habits are formed that help ensure that one continues to be healthy and well.

Practicing the Gluten Free Lifestyle

Back from the Brink — The Recovery of Good Health

Inez Castillo was a physical therapist working at a beautiful spa in Southern California. Her area of expertise focused on rehabilitation of athletic injuries. Inez was able to help her patients achieve rapid recovery from many exercise and sports related conditions, especially those involving ankle sprains or shoulder problems.

She loved her work, met interesting people, and was able to spend a lot of time in the golden California sunshine. She could schedule treatment sessions outdoors in the early morning and late afternoon when it wasn't too hot. In the middle of the day she worked in her indoor office, a large space with big windows. Earlier in her career, when she had been a physical therapist at a major New York City hospital, the view from her office was a dim, dusty, gray airshaft. After a few years of working in Manhattan, she had the opportunity to move to California. Inez didn't hesitate and soon built a wonderful new life for herself that made her happy. She had a glorious view of sepia-toned canyons spilling down a mountainside, framed by cactus, desert wildflowers, and a bright, pastel blue sky.

Inez always appreciated her good fortune in being able to live in Los Angeles County. The easy-going lifestyle and convenient access to the ocean, mountains, and desert suited her, and life was pretty much perfect until her life took a sudden left turn when her health deteriorated drastically within a few short days and she found herself desperately grasping for a lifeline.

She woke up on a clear, warm June morning gasping for breath. She couldn't swallow and felt like she couldn't breathe. By the time she arrived at the Emergency Department of Good Samaritan

Hospital her hands were red and her fingers had swelled to the size of sausages. All her tests came back normal and Inez was discharged, wondering what was happening to her.

During the next few months her hands remained red and swollen, and the skin began to crack open and bleed. She described the appearance as similar to a chemical burn. During September and October she developed upper respiratory allergies, as well as hives on her legs. An allergist prescribed a cortisone cream for the hives which failed to have any beneficial effect.

That winter Inez developed an allergic reaction in her eyes to her contact lenses and she contracted bronchitis, which was treated with antibiotics, but she had a severe allergic reaction to the medication, which required another Emergency Department visit to restore normal breathing.

Her health continued to deteriorate, but none of her physicians could identify a specific cause. Her allergies persisted and she became chronically fatigued and susceptible to the upper respiratory infections that she came in contact with, and she dreaded going to work where any of her patients could sneeze or cough in close proximity to her.

Polymyositis is an autoimmune disorder in which muscles are chronically inflamed. Symptoms include muscle weakness, pain, and possible loss of muscle mass around the shoulders and hips.

To make matters worse, her menstrual cycle ceased to function. It felt like all her body's systems were breaking down and she had lost all control over her health. She went to see a rheumatologist who ordered several different blood tests. Despite the fact that they were all normal, the doctor told her she had "mixed connective tissue disorder," an umbrella diagnosis for people with symptoms of lupus, scleroderma, and polymyositis. He prescribed Plaquenil, a drug primarily used to treat malaria and autoimmune diseases like lupus and rheumatoid arthritis. Plaquenil is described as a disease-modifying anti-rheumatic drug. Its mechanism of action involves reducing immunologic and inflammatory responses by interfering with cell-to-cell signaling. Its side effects include nausea, vomiting, heart problems, and eye toxicity, so Inez chose not to fill the prescription.

Still unwell a few months after her office visit, Inez saw another rheumatologist who specialized in nutritional disorders who did a variety of tests for food sensitivities. Inez learned she was malnourished, despite the fact that she was a healthy eater. She was low in essential amino acids, and zinc, and magnesium (important trace minerals) were undetectable in her body. She also had allergies to 21 different foods. In other words, Inez had multiple significant medical problems.

The doctor instructed her to eliminate all dairy products and all legumes from her diet, including eggs, which meant that she no longer had any vegetarian sources of protein. She did not eat meat and now had to rely on strictly vegan protein sources like nuts, seeds, broccoli, cauliflower, quinoa, and amaranth. The good news was that her symptoms improved dramatically. Her upper respiratory infections were less frequent, the hives on her legs occurred less, and the redness, swelling, and skin lesions on her hands were better.

The rheumatologist also prescribed vitamin and mineral supplementation in high doses, but after one year, Inez's blood levels of critical vitamins and minerals were barely within normal limits, despite popping lots of pills every day containing hundreds and thousands of times the recommended daily allowances. She continued to be sensitive to many foods, and wondered if any real progress had been made.

In addition, Inez continued to believe she had mixed connective tissue disorder. Believing she had a disease with aspects of both lupus and scleroderma created a great deal of anxiety and uncertainty about her future. She knew that those with lupus were in danger of developing additional life threatening conditions like kidney failure. She was also aware that people with scleroderma could develop serious complications affecting the heart and lungs. She didn't want to spend her days worrying about her health, but she knew she had real medical issues, but none of her doctors could solve her problems.

Her symptoms worsened during an office remodeling at her spa causing a severe skin reaction. She became profoundly fatigued and her face swelled so much she "looked like a toad" and the skin on her arms and legs was "triple-thick." Her muscles felt weak and she couldn't stand. A friend recommended she see yet another rheumatologist who appeared to have more insight. He performed an ELISA on Inez's blood, which showed she had antibodies to gluten.

Based on this result, he prescribed a gluten free diet.

> An **enzyme-linked immunosorbent assay (ELISA)** is a diagnostic test used to detect the presence of a specific antibody. The development of ELISA to detect anti-transglutaminase autoantibodies was a breakthrough in the diagnosis of celiac disease.

From Inez's point of view, going on a gluten free diet was a new recommendation. None of her other physicians had proposed such a diet and the recommendation was unwelcome. None of her doctors' prescriptions and recommendations resulted in any benefit, and going on a gluten free diet was more complicated than taking a pill or not eating dairy, eggs, and beans. She didn't want to begin anything that would take a lot of effort, considering that nothing seemed to work. She chose not to start this new diet, and instead took the Prednisone and Zyrtec he prescribed for her immune system problems and her allergies.

During the next year she continued to suffer. She "caught everybody's cold" and was always tired. She was very stressed and the fact that she couldn't do any exercise made her feel even more miserable. She did attend conferences, though, as she needed to keep her physical therapy license current. On a trip to San Diego to attend a weekend series of lectures on sports injury rehabilitation, she heard one of my presentations.

"Not another rheumatologist," she said to herself, but after my presentation she spoke with me about the interaction between food and performance, specifically referring to gluten intolerance as a common, although underdiagnosed, problem, and she decided to consult with us at our clinic. We ordered a new series of blood tests, including a panel of immunologic tests. One of them showed positive for HLA DQ8, which confirmed additional test results that suggested gluten intolerance. We told her that the primary culprit was gluten intolerance and recommended a gluten free diet.

She started it and noticed immediate benefits. One of the obvious changes was a large improvement in her energy levels. She was no longer tired and fatigued all day, every day and was no longer an easy target for any germ that came her way. Back in Manhattan she felt compelled to wash her hands if someone coughed or sneezed in her vicinity in an effort to ward off another round of infection and illness. On a gluten free diet, she didn't catch a cold or the flu for more than a year. The hives on her legs appeared once in a while, rather than frequently, and if she had dairy products like yogurt or cheese, her fingers only swelled a bit.

"I've got my immune system back," she said. Over time, she was able to cease all of her medications and her menstrual cycle returned to normal. She rarely gets sick, and returned to her normal weight, and now exercises regularly. In other words, she's a normal, healthy person. The turning point was starting the gluten free diet. Eliminating gluten was the key to solving the majority of her health issues.

The Gluten Free Manifesto

It's important to acknowledge that starting a gluten free diet is a major undertaking. When a doctor recommends that a patient adopt it, they usually stress that the diet is for life. There's no benefit to the patient if the doctor is reluctant to emphasize the stringency of this critical lifestyle change. When gluten intolerance is the primary cause of the person's problems, a life long gluten free diet is the primary solution. This news can be very tough to hear. But doctors know that such patients need to begin a gluten free program right away.

- Avoiding gluten is not the only important dietary goal for those who are gluten intolerant. Additional critical goals include:
- Getting enough quality protein, quality carbohydrate, and quality fat every day.
- Getting enough fruits and vegetables every day.
- Getting enough vitamins and minerals every day.
- Increasing "good" microorganisms and reducing "bad" microorganisms in the small intestine.
- Overcoming metabolic disease states (such as osteoporosis) caused by gluten intolerance and celiac disease.
- Restoring normal immune system functioning.

Normally, digestion is completed in the small intestine and nutrients are absorbed through the inner lining of the small intestine into the bloodstream. In **malabsorption syndrome**, many cells in this inner lining are defective, injured, or diseased, and nutrients aren't absorbed properly. Symptoms of malabsorption syndrome include diarrhea, abdominal cramps, abdominal bloating, weight loss, and swelling of the skin.

Malabsorption syndrome is often a consequence of being gluten intolerant. Many affected people have had various vitamin and mineral deficiencies for years in addition to being undernourished. It may seem to such people that they're eating enough, but owing to their gluten intolerance they haven't been able to absorb the nutrients they're consuming. Countering the effects of malabsorption syndrome is a primary goal for those recovering from disorders caused by gluten intolerance. All deficiencies must be addressed in the new gluten free diet for the patient to return to a normal healthy state.

The list of goals may seem lengthy, but many of these objectives are shared by everyone who wants to be healthy on an ongoing basis. The goals on the list become easy to accomplish once the actions involved become habitual. Reading nutrition labels and getting a realistic sense of your daily calorie consumption takes some time in the beginning, but these simple tasks quickly become second nature and fade into the background. The wonderful result is consuming enough quality food every day, getting the vitamins and minerals needed every day, successfully eliminating gluten from the diet and enjoying good health. All the unpleasant symptoms and problems are in the past, which restores the ability to live a full life again.

Tips for Starting a Gluten Free Diet

There are a lot of components involved in setting up a gluten free diet. The first part is learning which foods contain gluten, eliminating those and replacing them with gluten free items, but this is neither easy or as straightforward as it might seem. We'll discuss in detail how to accomplish the goal of replacing gluten containing foods in one's diet.

Those on a gluten free diet must not only avoid gluten, but also make sure the diet is nutritionally complete. Like every other person, they need to ensure they're getting enough protein, carbohydrate, and fat on a daily basis and need to consume enough total calories for their height and weight as well as taking the proper amounts of a broad spectrum of vitamins and minerals, which can be a challenge.

Until recently, most "gluten-free" foods on the market were devoid of quality nutrition. Most of them could be characterized as low nutrient density foods that they contained empty calories and not much more. People who are gluten intolerant need to consume gluten free foods that are high nutrient density products. A "gluten free" label may be a mere marketing ploy, and is not necessarily an indication that the product is going to be good for you.

Protein, Carbohydrates, and Fats

For those embarking on a gluten-free diet, it's important to understand their body's overall dietary requirements and to make sure they're meeting them. For example, a woman of average height and weight should consume approximately 1700 calories per day and a man of average height and weight should consume approximately 1800 calories per day.

A proper diet should consist of the following approximate percentages:

- Carbohydrates, 50%
- Proteins, 20%
- Fats, 30%

A gram of carbohydrate and a gram of protein each provide 4 calories of energy. A gram of fat provides 9 calories of energy. A woman on a 1700-calorie per day food plan should consume approximately 85 grams of protein, 210 grams of carbohydrate, and 60 grams of fat each day. A man on an 1800-calorie per day food plan should consume approximately 90 grams of protein, 225 grams of carbohydrate, and 60 grams of fat each day. These numbers are guidelines and not meant to be followed rigidly. If someone is malnourished they'll want to eat more of everything in proper proportions until they reach their target weight.

First we'll discuss the nutrients themselves and then talk about solving the special challenges involved in being on a gluten-free diet.

Protein

An important nutritional principle is to be sure to have a portion of protein at each meal. Whether man or a woman, a portion of protein is about the size of an open palm which translates into an approximate three-ounce portion of lean meat, lean poultry, or fish for a woman, and a four-ounce portion for a man. A four-ounce serving of salmon, tuna, or lean turkey contains approximately 25 grams of protein.

Why eat protein at every meal? The underlying principle here is food combining. The science behind food combining has been known for more than 40 years, but most fad diets and diet best sellers have forgotten about this key factor in healthy eating.

Food combining is critical to a normal, optimally functioning metabolism. When a person's metabolism is working efficiently they're using glucose (carbohydrate building blocks) instead of storing it. As a result, their blood insulin levels are steady throughout the day, rather than swinging wildly up and down, causing all kinds of internal havoc.

Insulin is a hormone produced by specialized cells in the pancreas. Insulin has many important functions, including causing muscle, liver, and fat cells to absorb glucose from the blood stream. An inability of the pancreas to produce sufficient insulin results in elevated blood glucose levels. This condition is known as type 1 diabetes.

Protein is necessary for the proper use of the carbohydrates we eat. Without protein to slow carbohydrate digestion, sugars get dumped into the bloodstream and blood insulin levels spike. High insulin concentrations cause glucose to be rapidly absorbed by muscle and fat cells, and blood glucose levels plummet, then rise again when we eat the next high carbohydrate meal. Our bodies are literally riding a rollercoaster, and our mental processes are experiencing similar jolts.

Eventually, the glucose rollercoaster causes a person to become resistant to insulin, resulting in a pre-diabetic state. If their dietary habits are not remedied, diabetes is often the long-term outcome. For a person who is gluten intolerant, cyclical glucose spiking creates additional physiologic pressure. The necessary first corrective step is to add protein to every meal, which regulates how glucose is absorbed and used.

The benefits of food combining are wide ranging, including a human performance benefit. Eating balanced meals helps our brains work better. Food combining helps us think much more clearly and more creatively. Food combining also eliminates that late afternoon burned-out feeling which is your body's way of saying, "Stop, I can't take it any more." That 4:00 p.m. sleep-inducing crash is caused by the extreme insulin and glucose swings a person has experienced all day long. Combining protein with carbohydrate at every meal is a simple and straightforward means of beginning to resolve these issues.

Carbohydrates

Complex carbohydrates are chains of three or more sugar molecules. Grains, pastas, root vegetables, beans and lentils, corn, apples, berries, and pears are excellent sources of complex carbohydrates. Digestion of complex carbohydrates into simple sugar molecules is a slow process. In food, simple sugars consist of individual molecules of glucose, fructose, and sucrose. Simple sugars are quickly digested and absorbed into the bloodstream.

It's best to consume complex carbohydrates and avoid simple carbohydrates whenever possible. The word carbohydrate means the molecule is composed of carbon, hydrogen, and oxygen. Sugar molecules are the building blocks of carbohydrates. When we eat foods that contain a lot of simple sugars like sugar itself, cookies, cake, candy, and soda, the sugar (glucose) doesn't need to be digested. It's already in its simplest form and goes right into the bloodstream. Insulin is released from the pancreas and the glucose is transported either to tissues that need it for energy or to regions of fat cells where it's converted to fat. When you eat simple sugars your body cannot regulate how much glucose is absorbed at a time. Usually more glucose becomes available than the amount needed for energy, and the excess is stored as fat.

Eating complex carbohydrates enables the body to use glucose for energy steadily over the course of the day. Digesting complex carbohydrates takes time. Glucose is absorbed slowly, and more of it is used for energy. Complex carbohydrates are an excellent source of energy. Consumed in the right proportions, complex carbohydrates will rarely be converted into fat. Simple sugars on the other hand are readily processed into fat and provide excess levels of energy at inappropriate intervals. The best the body can do is store this energy as fat.

How much is a portion of complex carbohydrates? Once again, the natural world provides a convenient and effective solution. One apple, one orange, or one pear each comprises a portion of complex carbohydrates. A bunch of grapes the size of your fist is a portion. One sweet potato, two big carrots, a cup of squash, each of these is a portion of complex carbohydrates. One half cup of beans or lentils is a portion. One slice of bread is a portion. Basically, a portion of complex carbohydrates represents 100 calories of energy.

Fats

Fats have mistakenly gotten a bad reputation during the last 30 or 40 years. Oversimplification and factual errors led to a series of media-driven misconceptions. First, everyone was told cholesterol is bad for you, then cholesterol was good. Next there were different kinds of cholesterol. Some were bad and some were good. Eggs were bad. As of this writing, the "right kinds" of eggs are good. Butter was bad, then it was okay, then butter was bad again because it contained small amounts of trans-fat. This carousel of conflicting recommendations has damaged consumer confidence in federal agencies responsible for public health recommendations.

Fats are an important part of every person's diet. These nutrients are a major source of energy, as well as being a critical component of almost every cell in the body. Fats are the main constituent of the cell membrane, the outer "smart" lining that lets in materials needed by the cell, keeps out those materials which are not wanted, and allows waste products to be transported out of the cell.

Fats are used in the construction of specialized tissues such as the brain, spinal cord, and nerves. They help cushion and protect nerve bundles and help speed up transmission of electrical signals. In addition, fats help regulate body temperature and cushion and protect organs like the heart, liver, and pancreas. Basically, fats are necessary for life, so fats are not the problem.

Too much fat is a problem, and too much saturated fat is a big problem. Saturated fats are found in palm oil, coconut oil, chocolate, butter, cream, and cheese, as well as in certain meats. High concentrations of saturated fat result in solid, rather than liquid, substances. Butter and margarine, for example, contain high concentrations of saturated fat.

"Saturated" is a description of the structure of the fat molecule that consists of a series of single electrochemical bonds connecting the various atoms filling all the bonding positions. Unsaturated fat molecules contain various amounts of double or even triple bonds, and many connecting positions have yet to be filled. These double and triple bonds contain energy that your body can use for its own metabolic purposes. Saturated fats cannot be used for energy. All your body can do with saturated fats is store them in fat cells or deposit them in places where they don't belong, like in the walls of blood vessels.

How much fat should a person consume each day? Depending on height and weight, approximately 60 grams of fat per day is a good average. Individual needs will vary and if an individual finds they're gaining weight or their waistline has expanded, reduce daily fat intake by 10 grams. This modification should bring things back to normal.

The Gluten Free Diet

Now that we have a good general nutritional background, we can talk about the specifics of a gluten free diet. First we'll discuss foods to include, then we'll look at foods to avoid, and finally we'll consider foods of which we should be suspicious of.

Foods to Include

A gluten free diet doesn't have to be a highly restricted, monotonous diet. There are plenty of healthy, delicious, and nutritious choices available, and there's no need to feel deprived or bored. It's important to eliminate all sources of gluten from your diet, but once that's done there's an almost unlimited variety of interesting foods to choose from. The main categories include:

- Fats
- Fruits
- Grains
- Proteins
- Spices
- Vegetables

Proteins for Gluten Intolerant People

There is an abundance of protein sources with plenty of variety available for those who eat meat, as well as for those who are vegetarians. High-quality protein foods include:

- Beans and lentils
- Chicken
- Eggs
- Lamb
- Lean beef
- Lean turkey
- Low-fat cheese
- Low-fat yogurt
- Milk
- Salmon
- Tuna

It is important to get complete protein every day. It is provided by a food or combination of foods that contains all 20 amino acids which are the building blocks of protein. Our bodies can manufacture 12 of these building blocks, but we have to obtain the remaining eight from the food we eat. These eight building blocks are known as "essential amino acids."

Complete protein is found in red meat, turkey, chicken, fish, eggs, milk, cheese, yogurt, and avocados. Those on a vegetarian diet that contains neither dairy products or eggs need to be sure they're obtaining complete protein. Beans and lentils are good sources, but these foods do not contain all the necessary amino acids. Avocados are a delicious source of complete protein. Amaranth, buckwheat, and quinoa are grains that provide complete protein and are critically important for vegans. Also, combining legumes, grains, nuts, and seeds at various meals ensures a diet that contains all the essential amino acids.

Carbohydrates

A wide variety of whole foods are excellent sources of complex carbohydrates, including the following fruits, vegetables, legumes, and grains:

Fruits
- Apples
- Apricots
- Grapefruit
- Grapes
- Oranges
- Pears
- Plums
- Strawberries

Vegetables
- Carrots
- Corn
- Squash
- Sweet potatoes

Legumes

- Beans
- Lentils
- Split peas

Whole grains and grain-like crops (non-gluten-containing)

- Amaranth
- Brown rice
- Buckwheat
- Millet
- Quinoa
- Red rice
- Teff
- Wild rice

Combining complex carbohydrates with protein in a series of small meals throughout the day provides the body with a steady, consistent source of energy. Protein provides the building blocks for construction of new materials, cells and tissues, and carbohydrates provide the energy needed for these construction activities.

The grains and grain-like foods in a gluten free diet are not usually found in a supermarket's bread department. A little legwork is needed to track down stores and chains that carry gluten free grains and breads. The good news is that many local markets and national chains are discovering that gluten free foods are a large niche. Proprietors are learning that many people are searching for reliable sources of gluten free foods.

Quinoa is a grain-like crop that has been grown in the South American Andean region for more than 5,000 years. It has a light, fluffy texture, a mild nutty taste, and can be substituted for rice, millet, or couscous in any recipe. When combined with beans, lentils, or split peas, quinoa is terrific in stews, pilafs, and casseroles. It can also be purchased in the form of breakfast flakes, similar to corn flakes.

Like quinoa, amaranth is a grain-like plant. It is a traditional food in Africa and is grown in Asia and the Americas. As part of a gluten free diet, amaranth seeds can be combined with dried fruit, nuts, and other seeds in breakfast muesli, or puffed amaranth can be eaten as a breakfast cereal. Cooked amaranth can be added to omelets or salads.

The millets are a group of small seeded grains which are gluten free and sources of complete protein. These grains have a mild nutty flavor and go well with tahini and other nut butters. Millet is also delicious when combined with raisins, dried fruit, almonds, and oranges. From a vegetable perspective, millet goes well with black beans, lentils, mushrooms, and squash.

Teff is a grass native to northeastern Africa. Its seeds are the smallest grains in the world. It is highly nutritious, containing complete protein and abundant carbohydrates (25 grams per half-cup). Teff flour is an excellent ingredient for baking quick breads because of its slightly gelatinous texture. Teff flour and rice flour can be combined in all sorts of delicious muffin and desert bread recipes.

Buckwheat is another highly nutritious grain-like plant that is related to rhubarb. Diets containing buckwheat have been linked to reduced risks of heart disease and high blood pressure. Buckwheat soba noodles are a traditional Japanese dish. (Make sure the soba noodles do not contain wheat as an additive.) Buckwheat flour has a strong nutty taste and makes wonderful pancakes. Buckwheat groats are the whole or raw buckwheat kernel used in kasha, a staple in families of Eastern European heritage.

More good news: there are plenty of gluten free pastas available. These delicious pastas are made from brown rice, quinoa, amaranth, and corn. Gluten-free pastas are available in many shapes and sizes, including penne, shells, linguine, fusilli, and lasagna sheets. When buying gluten-free pasta, it's important to be familiar with the manufacturer, making sure the pasta is made in dedicated gluten free facilities. When in doubt, call the manufacturer for detailed information.

Fats

The largest proportion of fats in any diet, gluten free or otherwise, should derive from monounsaturated and polyunsaturated fats. All the high-energy bonds in saturated fats have already been occupied (saturated), so these fats are not efficient sources of energy, so our bodies store them. Saturated fats are the main dietary factors in raising blood cholesterol levels. Elevated blood cholesterol leads to fat deposits in the walls of arteries, resulting in high blood pressure and heart disease.

Healthy fats, monounsaturated and polyunsaturated fat, are found in many of the following gluten-free foods:

- Avocados
- Nuts
- Seeds
- Canola oil
- Olive oil
- Peanut oil
- Safflower oil
- Sesame seed oil
- Sunflower seed oil

In the small intestine, fat digestion produces fatty acids, the building blocks of dietary fat. Omega-3 fatty acids are a specific type of polyunsaturated fat that is beneficial in reducing the risk of heart disease and related conditions. Omega-3 fatty acids help reduce blood pressure and help protect the heart by lowering the risk of coronary artery disease. Omega-3 fatty acids also help protect against several types of cancer and boost immune function.

Excellent dietary sources of omega-3 fatty acids include the following:

- Flax seed oil and flax seeds
- Salmon
- Sardines
- Walnuts

Flax seed oil can be purchased in health food stores and markets. One tablespoon ensures the daily requirement for omega-3 fatty acids.

Fruits and Vegetables

Fruits and vegetables are an important component of any diet and are especially important in gluten free diets. "Five To Stay Alive" is the promotional tag line many national organizations have been using to raise public consciousness about the need to eat fresh fruits and vegetables every day. Most of us blissfully ignore this important dietary recommendation. When we're standing at the open refrigerator door at 10 p.m., thinking about a late night snack, we're not really looking for a nice carrot, broccoli floret, or crunchy pear. We're looking for leftover cake.

If a sweet tooth rules the majority of food decisions, whether gluten intolerant or not, it means trouble. In contrast, the life-long health benefits provided by eating fresh fruits and vegetables are substantial. It's important to keep reminding people to make sure they eat enough fruits and vegetables every day.

What makes fruits and vegetables nutritional mainstays, and why are they so important to good health and long life? First, fruits and vegetables are excellent sources of vitamins and minerals. What most people don't know, and what nutritional science isn't even close to figuring out, is how vitamins and minerals combine in the body and work together to provide optimal health.

Recommended daily allowances of vitamins and minerals have been calculated long ago, and many already know that calcium and vitamin D work together. They also know that B vitamins are important for proper nerve system functioning, and that vitamin C helps strengthen the immune system. We know a little about how vitamins and minerals work, but we don't know a lot. We certainly don't know how to put specific quantities of vitamins and minerals together so a person obtains what's needed to be healthy, but we don't have to do these calculations. Nature has already done this for us.

The vitamins and minerals we need are available in the right quantities and the right combinations at our local market. All we have to do is buy them, prepare them, and eat enough of them every day. National organizations have determined that five daily portions of fresh fruits and vegetables are necessary for everyone. You can eat more, but eating less is not in your best interests.

Which five to eat? The optimal recommendation is a wide variety, the more colorful, the better. If a plate has something red, green, orange or yellow on it, it's a good selsection. Nature has already put the vitamins and minerals needed into fruits and vegetables. It's up to us to do our job and eat them.

In addition to providing necessary vitamins and minerals, fruits and vegetables are packed with phytonutrients. "Phyto" is derived from a Greek word meaning "plant." Phytonutrients are biochemicals that perform a broad range of health maintaining and health improving functions. Hundreds of phytonutrients have been isolated and identified, and tens of thousands of varieties are yet to be discovered.

Many phytonutrients are powerful antioxidants, others help prevent chronic diseases like cancer and heart disease, and others help improve immune system functioning, but you can't get your daily dose of phytonutrients in a pill or capsule. They need to be obtained naturally. These biochemicals occur in various combinations that need to be intact for the phytonutrients to work at all. Each one has a specific role to play, and different fruits and vegetables contain different varieties.

Brightly colored fruits and vegetables contain high concentrations of powerful phytonutrients, another important reason for consuming a variety of these foods. The more a plate or salad bowl resembles an artist's palette, the more healthful the meal will be.

Foods to Avoid

Those who are gluten intolerant should avoid all breads, cookies, cakes, muffins, biscuits, pastas, pizza, and bagels that contain wheat, barley, and rye, which are the primary gluten containing grains consumed in the West. The main challenge for people eating gluten free is that wheat, barley, and rye are everywhere.

Some foods are hidden sources of gluten. It's common for a gluten intolerant person to be on a gluten free diet and continue to have persistent symptoms. The person is not only still unwell, but they become discouraged and frustrated with themselves and their doctor, thinking that they're doing the right thing. They haven't eaten a bagel, a slice of pizza, or a cheese Danish in many months, so why does their stomach still hurt and why do they still have unpleasant intestinal problems?

The answer is that if someone is gluten intolerant, even trace amounts can provoke a full range of symptoms. A product may not list gluten among its ingredients but the manufacturing process may have employed machinery and utensils that have been in contact with gluten. Grains of gluten can contaminate the final product and the result is food that is not gluten free. Vitamin supplements and pharmaceuticals present the same problem. Those who aren't specialists would never think that a pill or tablet could contain gluten, but medicines and supplements in pill and tablet form often contain sufficient gluten to cause substantial problems for gluten intolerant persons. The active ingredients may be gluten free, but the filler and stabilizers may contain gluten, or the manufacturing process introduces gluten. In either case, such pills cause symptoms in a gluten intolerant person who thinks they are on a gluten-free diet. These hidden sources of gluten are more than frustrating. They represent actual threats to the gluten intolerant person's health and welfare.

How much gluten contamination is too much? Less than 20 parts per million (ppm; a standard measure of concentration) can provoke symptoms in a gluten intolerant person. Some oat containing foods that are labeled "gluten free" have been shown to contain 400 ppm! Buyer beware is the watchword when you're gluten intolerant.

A major piece of the puzzle is to ensure that your gluten free diet is actually free of gluten. This takes some work, but for affected individuals the rewards are great in terms of good health. As they gain experience, they learn which foods to include, which to avoid, and which to be suspicious of. A gluten free diet is dynamic, not static, and involves a lot of experimentation. The gluten free concept has begun to penetrate the food industry's consciousness, and new products are coming to market all the time. The key is to learn which manufacturers are trustworthy and which products meet the high standards required by those who are gluten intolerant. As mentioned in Chapter 3, companies that have earned gluten free certification from either the Celiac Support Association or the Gluten Intolerance Group are listed on their websites (csaceliacs.org and gfco.org)

Oats are a special consideration. Although they do not contain gluten, often the facilities where they are processed can contaminate the oats with wheat flour. In addition, oats may be contaminated on a farm by adjacent fields of wheat, barley, or rye. They can be a valuable dietary component for those who are gluten intolerant as an important ingredient in breads as well as a good source of protein, but caution is necessary.

Some people with celiac disease may be sensitive to oats and develop symptoms after eating food that contains oats. In such cases, the person's body is producing antibodies against specific oat proteins, a reaction that might be related to an overall heightened immune response. Generally, people beginning a gluten free diet should maintain three months of being gluten free before introducing a small amount of oats. Living gluten free for three months greatly reduces the load on one's immune system and may make it easier to tolerate oats. If they can be consumed without provoking a reaction, then one's dietary possibilities have expanded.

The following grains and related products should be avoided by gluten intolerant people at all times:

- Bulgur
- Couscous
- Farro
- Orzo
- Seitan
- Soba (except when made from buckwheat)
- Spelt
- Tabouli
- Tempeh
- Triticale
- Udon

Most of the items on this list are staples in the whole grains sections of health food stores and served on the menus of many vegetarian and vegan restaurants, but all of them are grains in the wheat family or are made from wheat.

Spelt (*Triticum spelta*) is often described as being gluten-free, but it is closely related to common wheat (*Triticum aestivim*) and contains a moderate amount of gluten. Triticale is a hybrid of wheat and rye. Farro is an Italian term that describes three different types of wheat, (*Triticum dicoccon*), einkorn (*Triticum monococcom*), and spelt.

Bulgur is made from several different wheat species and is a staple of Middle Eastern, Mediterranean, and Indian cuisine. Couscous consists of spherical granules of grain made from semolina wheat. Couscous is a staple of North African and Middle Eastern cooking. Orzo is rice-shaped pasta made from semolina wheat.

Tempeh originated in Indonesia and is a vegetarian substitute for meat made primarily from soybeans, but may contain wheat and barley. Tabouli is a spicy vegetable-and-grain dish that originated in the Middle East. The grain component is bulgur. Seitan is made from gluten and is served in vegetarian and vegan restaurants. It originated as a dish in Japan, China, and Southeast Asia. Soba are thin noodles made from buckwheat, but many manufacturers add wheat. Udon are thick noodles made from wheat. Both soba and udon originated in Japan.

Additional Foods with Hidden Gluten

Many additional foods contain wheat, but we don't usually think of them as breads or grains, and we don't suspect we're consuming gluten when we eat or drink them. A short list includes:

- Beer
- Brewer's yeast
- Brown rice syrup
- Licorice
- Malt
- Malt vinegar
- Potato chips
- Soy sauce
- Processed foods
- Bread crumbs
- Deli meat
- Fish cakes
- Frozen burgers
- Sausage

Brown rice syrup is an especially tricky food. People think that because it is derived from brown rice, it must be gluten free, but the base for the syrup contains wheat. Malts are primarily derived from barley, so beer, malted milk, and malt vinegar need to be avoided by anyone on a gluten free diet. The good news is that gluten free beer exists and these beers are often made from buckwheat or sorghum. There are dozens of delicious gluten free beers manufactured by craft breweries, and the first International Gluten Free Beer Festival was held in 2006 in the United Kingdom!

Soy sauce is also off limits because the base contains wheat. The primary ingredient in licorice is wheat and gluten is one of the main ingredients in brewer's yeast. Wheat is often an ingredient in processed foods that provides bulk and serves as a base.

Reading the label is the key to guarding against unwanted sources of gluten. The U.S. Food and Drug Administration (FDA) has compiled the Major Food Allergens List, a list of the top eight allergens which account for 90% of food allergy reactions. Wheat is number seven on the list which also includes milk, eggs, fish, nuts, and soybeans.

Our concern isn't being allergic to wheat as such. Gluten intolerance is a result of an immune system response, which is distinct physiologically from an allergic reaction. Those with a wheat allergy might experience an itchy rash, hives, asthma, or symptoms of hay fever. Gluten intolerance (and celiac disease) is a multisystem disorder usually involving destructive changes to the small intestine and possible associated autoimmune diseases, but those who are gluten intolerant benefit from the FDA's list, as the 2004 Food Allergen Labeling and Consumer Protection Act requires that food labels clearly identify any food sources or ingredients that are on, or are derived from the Major Food Allergens list.

Foods to Question

Many additional foods do not contain wheat as a main ingredient, but are questionable in that wheat may be used as filler or to provide bulk to a sauce or liquid. These foods include:

- Condiments
- Fried foods
- Salad dressings
- Sauces
- Soups

Condiments like mustard can contain wheat flour. Sauces can contain wheat based starch as a filler and binder. Salad dressings can contain malt vinegar (malt is made from barley). Soups, whether canned or dried, can contain wheat starch or hydrolyzed wheat protein. Snacks and fried foods can be prepared with gluten containing oils. Read the labels. If the product contains wheat, the label must list it to be in compliance with the Food Allergen Labeling and Consumer Protection Act.

Be suspicious whenever a label lists "natural flavors". They can contain hidden gluten. If the label lists all the ingredients, none of which are wheat, barley, or rye, you're probably on safe ground. Learning how to read labels is a key life skill for those who are gluten intolerant. Who would think that a dairy product contains gluten? It's dairy, but soft cheeses and grated cheese may contain breadcrumbs or wheat flour based seasonings. Seasoning packets are another potential danger zone that can contain wheat, wheat starch, or soy sauce.

How to Begin a Gluten Free Diet

When someone is told to go on a gluten free diet, it can feel like being told they have to go on a difficult, possibly perilous journey. They don't want to do it, and may think they can't possibly succeed even if they convince themselves to try, but once they begin, they may find it well worth the effort.

It's important to have a successful launch to new gluten free circumstances, and symptomatic setbacks will be discouraging and stressful. As so many packaged foods in cans, boxes, and jars, contain hidden gluten, it's best to avoid all packaged and processed food at the beginning of a gluten-free diet. A successful gluten free diet begins with fresh whole foods. Here's a short general list:

- Eggs
- Fresh or frozen fish
- Fresh fruits and vegetables
- Fresh turkey, chicken, and lean meat
- Milk, yogurt, and non-processed cheese
- Whole grain gluten free breads

Vegetarians should leave out the foods that aren't on their regular list and need to make sure they get complete protein every day. The goal is to have successful food experiences every day, and eating only fresh whole foods will ensure this daily goal.

Ninety continuous days of eating only fresh whole foods establishes a powerful benchmark. During these three months, no gluten has reached the small intestines, and as a result there are no adverse immunologic responses. The chronic inflammation of the small intestine has likely been considerably reduced, and the immune system is no longer on perpetual high alert. Many longstanding symptoms have probably begun to decrease and recede. The reduction in symptoms is, of course, a very potent motivating factor for continuing on this new life path.

Once on a gluten free diet for three months it's okay to experiment a little. Try bread made from oats that is labeled gluten free. If there's gluten contamination there might be a mild reaction, but probably a less severe one than not being gluten free for the previous three months. If there are no symptoms after eating the oat bread, something new and interesting has been added to the diet!

Next, try a gluten free packaged pizza and see whether it's okay, gluten free ice cream in a gluten free ice cream cone. or gluten free biscuits made from a packaged mix. Not all at once, of course. If being on a gluten free diet works and a person can actually do what's needed to be on the diet, then they can try new foods and discover whether they can add them to their expanding list of safe and healthy foods.

Our list of fresh whole foods could be followed with infinite variety for a long time, and after a while you might not even want to eat food that comes in a box or can.

Why not make your own food and avoid foods that are processed and packaged? Some manufacturers do make nutritious and healthful products. In general, packaged and processed foods contain too much salt, too much sugar, and too much fat. Reading the labels on processed meats and processed dairy products will reveal lengthy paragraphs listing chemicals, additives, and stabilizers. None of these are healthy and none of them are actually food and should not intentionally be included in anyone's diet.

For those who are gluten intolerant, cooking their own food has the important benefit of avoiding packaged foods that may contain trace or even significant amounts of gluten. By making their own food, they can save time reading labels to make sure the products and packages are gluten free and they can save time calling manufacturers who haven't listed all their ingredients to avoid unpleasant surprises when a supposedly gluten free package or processed food turns out to include trace amounts of gluten. For someone who is gluten intolerant, being on a gluten free diet is beneficial in many respects. Not only are they helping themselves recover from a life-long set of health problems, but they're also eating much more nutritious food daily. In addition, they're not eating anything that isn't good for them. They're eating fresh whole foods packed with vitamins, minerals, and phytonutrients. Their meals are naturally balanced and they're consuming the right amounts of protein, carbohydrates, and fats, they sleep better and feel more rested. They have more strength to do vigorous exercise, and people begin to notice their healthy glow. All in all, life is good.

Being Gluten Free in a Family Setting

If an entire family or household is gluten intolerant, converting the kitchen into one big gluten free zone is straightforward. Eliminating the contaminants can take some time, but after this has been accomplished it's basically done. If only some family members are gluten intolerant, then a number of action steps to implement to avoid gluten cross contamination, including:

- Designating a gluten-free section of the kitchen
- Using separate blenders
- Using separate cutting boards
- Using separate spreads
- Using separate toasters

Eliminating the contaminants does require diligence and some creativity. Go through the refrigerator and throw out everything suspected of containing gluten, then take everything that's left out of the refrigerator and clean it thoroughly. Do the same with kitchen cabinets. Wash all the dishes, silverware, and utensils in hot, soapy water and make sure they're clean. Next, take a selection of dishware and store them in the new gluten free kitchen area, only to be used by those who on a gluten free diet.

Be sure to have separate toasters, blenders, and cutting boards for family members who are gluten free. Even a single breadcrumb can contain enough gluten to send an intolerant person over the edge, so the one-time expense of adding duplicate appliances and cooking tools is money well spent. Some kitchen utensils and tools are porous and retain specks of gluten-containing food, even after they've been thoroughly cleaned. Old cutting boards, ladles, and spatulas are to be used only by those not on a gluten free diet.

Usually a family shares jars of peanut butter, jam, mayonnaise, and mustard. Knives, spoons, and even forks go from the jar to the slice of bread and back to the jar. This won't work for the person who is gluten free, so separate jars clearly labeled "gluten free" need to be available and only used by those on a gluten free diet.

These tasks sound like a lot of work, but how they are approached will make all the difference in effectiveness and, ultimately, in health and happiness. Proactively choosing to accomplish these tasks is a powerful, positive attitude, as opposed to the disempowering attitude of "I have to do it." Choosing to do each job completely and having fun while doing it will help focus on what's being done and why, good health for everyone in the family.

Guess Who's Coming to Dinner?

House guests are often a challenge for a gluten free household. Most guests are unfamiliar with the rhythms and routines of a gluten free life and are unaware of the practice of using separate utensils for gluten containing foods, and unaware that the knife they've used to spread tahini on a whole-wheat pita should not be placed next to a plate of gluten free person.

We want our guests to enjoy themselves and mistakes will be made, although we don't want to draw attention to our guests' unintentional and innocent miscues. It's a good idea to inform your friends in advance of your gluten free concerns.

Dinner Reservations and Reservations About Dinner

For the gluten intolerant, eating out involves a certain level of risk taking and a leap of faith. Unless you're going to a restaurant that has a dedicated gluten-free menu, and you have gluten intolerant friends who've eaten there successfully, there's always an element of the unknown.

There are a number of strategies that go far toward ensuring an enjoyable night out. Knowing in advance where you're dining and being aware of the gluten free options on the menu is helpful. Calling ahead of time and speaking with the manager or chef can help to learn whether the restaurant can accommodate the needed dietary requirements.

It may be possible to address some areas of concern. For example, if the restaurant doesn't have a dedicated gluten free grill, could your salmon or tuna or chicken be grilled in its own foil wrapper?

Many natural food restaurants have a wide selection of gluten free dishes and are experienced in serving customers with a high level of food consciousness. Most places, though, represent a roll of the dice. Again, once you've succeeded in achieving your first three months of being gluten free, you may be able to better tolerate something unexpected. For the most part, it's well worth taking the time to find those restaurants that have authentic gluten free menus and are known to the gluten free community.

Beyond Gluten Free: When a Gluten Free Diet Isn't Enough

Gluten Intolerance, Celiac Disease, and Associated Disorders

Being on a gluten free diet itself may not relieve all symptoms. A person can be following a strict gluten free diet and continue experiencing persistent symptoms associated with any of the following conditions:

- Diamine oxidase deficiency and food allergies
- Endocrine problems
- Intolerance to foods that are cross-reactive with gluten
- Leaky gut syndrome
- Malabsorption and nutrient deficiencies
- Prolamine intolerance
- Yeast in the gut

Celiac disease is characterized as a chronic inflammatory disorder caused by an inappropriate immune response of intestinal T cells to gluten peptides and similar prolamine peptides (See Chapter 2). These peptides are rendered more immunogenic following deamidation by tissue transglutaminase. Gluten and prolamine peptides form antigen–antibody complexes with HLA-DQ2 or HLA-DQ8 proteins which are presented to intestinal T cells, initiating an immune reaction and inflammatory response. Gluten-reactive intestinal T cells are identified in virtually all patients with celiac disease, but not in normal individuals.

For many people who are gluten intolerant, and certainly for those affected by celiac disease, adhering to a strict gluten free diet is a key component of maintaining good health. If a patient is gluten intolerant and doesn't experience additional clinical issues, they can expect to feel better after 3–6 months of a strict gluten free diet, but clinical experience shows that up to 70% of patients with gluten intolerance have additional problems. For those with associated disorders such as yeast infections or gluten cross-reactivity, it can take up to a year of a strict gluten free diet to feel better.

Malabsorption and Nutrient Deficiencies

Malabsorption is caused by numerous conditions including celiac disease, alterations in the normal composition of the intestinal microbiome (dysbiosis), absence or low levels of digestive enzymes, chronic pancreatitis, and parasite infection. It can be evaluated by blood tests focused on nutrient deficiencies.

Malabsorption can cause deficiencies in vitamin B12, vitamin D, biotin, zinc, copper, iron, and magnesium, as well as elevated homocysteine levels. Vitamin B12 deficiency is associated with fatigue, brain fog, and pernicious anemia. Vitamin D deficiency is associated with muscle cramps, deposition of calcium in joints (pseudogout), and osteoporosis. Biotin deficiency is associated with hair loss and brittle nails, circumstances that are commonly found in persons with gluten intolerance and celiac disease. Zinc and copper deficiencies are associated with eye dryness, poor healing of wounds, and abnormal liver function. Magnesium deficiency is associated with constipation, muscle cramps, and leg cramps.

Elevated homocysteine represents a disturbance in methylation pathways. Homocysteine is a sulfur-containing amino acid whose methylation (a biochemical process requiring vitamin B12) creates the amino acid, methionine. Accumulation of homocysteine (for example, secondary to vitamin B12 deficiency or a mutation in the methylenetetrahydrofolate reductase [MTHFR] gene) strongly inhibits all methylation reactions. Defective methylation is associated with cardiovascular disease such as arteriosclerosis, heart attack, and stroke, diabetes, chronic inflammation, fatigue, and mood disorders like anxiety, panic attacks, and depression.

Treatment of Malabsorption Disorders

Many of the clinical disorders associated with malabsorption are alleviated or remedied by specific methods of dietary supplementation, including:

- Betaine HCl for insufficient production of gastric hydrochloric acid
- Digestive enzymes for pancreatic insufficiency and deficient production of pancreatic digestive enzymes
- Methyl folate, trimethylglycine, and methyl B12 for methylation defects
- Milk thistle to normalize bile chemical composition
- Ox bile to activate digestive enzymes
- Probiotics and prebiotics for alterations in the intestinal microbiome (dysbiosis)
- Vitamin B12 for pernicious anemia

Vitamin B12 is susceptible to breakdown by acidic pH and digestive enzymes, so it is given by injection or sublingual capsules. Defective methylation pathways, related to specific genetic mutations (such as MTHFR mutation) or elevated homocysteine levels, are easily correctable in 70–80% of patients with appropriate supplementation. Dysbiosis is easily correctable by supplementation with probiotics and prebiotics in up to 100% of patients with gluten intolerance and celiac disease. Supplementation with probiotics promotes restoration of the normal composition of the commensal microbiome and homeostasis of these microbial populations while prebiotics stimulate the growth and development of helpful symbiotic intestinal microorganisms.

Yeast in the Gut

Candida albicans is the most common human fungal pathogen. Normally, *C. albicans* is a harmless commensal microorganism, but it is opportunistic and its overgrowth leads to various pathologies in the host. In conditions of intestinal microbiome homeostasis, yeast overgrowth is controlled by other microorganisms, however in dysbiosis, yeast growth is unchecked and symptoms of yeast infection develop. The pathological presence of yeast in the gastrointestinal (GI) tract results from a vicious cycle that typically begins with an infection. The patient takes antibiotics, which destroy "friendly" (commensal) symbiotic GI bacteria, and *Candida albicans* spreads opportunistically in the GI tract where it secretes toxins that provoke an inflammatory response and weaken the immune system. The patient's compromised immune system enables the spread of another infection, and the vicious cycle repeats.

Problems begin when the yeast life cycle process transforms round, unicellular forms into budding, multicellular forms (hyphae). This transformation impacts the pathogenic potential of *C. albicans*. The Candida round form is benign and helpful to host physiology, but the hyphal form is more invasive and linked to the expression of Candida genes encoding virulence factors. Toxin expression stimulates the host immune system and provokes an inflammatory response. Yeast overgrowth leads to increased production of metabolites, which further provoke the host inflammatory response. Expanding *C. albicans* colonies form biofilms consisting of a dense network of round forms, hyphae, and pseudohyphae. The complex three-dimensional biofilm structure enables it to resist environmental changes and makes yeast difficult to eradicate. The biofilm lifestyle leads to dramatically increased protection from host defenses and increased levels of resistance to commonly used antibiotics and antifungal agents.

The presence of yeast in the GI tract is demonstrated by various symptoms including a craving for sweets, abdominal bloating, postprandial fatigue, migraine headaches, acne, hives, and eczema. Its treatment focuses on controlling yeast overgrowth by reducing the yeast count (the quantity of yeast microorganisms in the intestinal tract), preventing hyphae and biofilm formation. Yeasts thrive on carbohydrates and practical solutions for yeast infections begin with methods that deny nutrition to Candida colonies. A low carbohydrate diet and supplementation with digestive enzymes and betaine HCl (facilitating host digestion) will normalize colonies of helpful microorganisms and deny nutrition to yeast. Supplementation with probiotics and prebiotics acts to reverse dysbiosis and normalize the gastrointestinal microbiome. Reducing quantities of yeast in the GI tract is accomplished by supplementation with Candidacillin, pau d'arco (*Tabebuia avellanedae*), Artemisia plus berberine, and black walnut hulls.

Candidacillin is a proprietary blend of four food ingredients that act to optimize the intestinal microbiome and control intestinal yeast overgrowth by preventing yeast hyphae and biofilm formation. Candidacillin contains calcium undecylate (the calcium salt of undecylic acid is FDA approved to treat Candida infections), caprylic acid, monolaurine, and calcium disodium EDTA. Calcium undecylate is derived from castor oil and inhibits conversion of yeast round cells into pathogenic filamentous hyphae. It is an antifungal agent that kills yeast cells. Caprylic acid (octanoic acid) is found in the milk of various mammals and in coconut oil. It possesses strong antimicrobial and antifungal activity and inhibits growth of *C. albicans*, *Staphylococcus aureus*, and various strains of streptococci. Monolaurine (glycerol monolaurate) is also found in coconut oil and human breast milk. Monolaurine has strong antimicrobial and antifungal activity, which is amplified by EDTA, a chelating agent that binds heavy metals. It also acts to destroy biofilms and kills yeast. Compliance with a Candidacillin treatment protocol results in a 90–95% success rate.

Yeast Infection (Candidiasis) Self-Assessment

1. Do you have a craving for sugar/sweets?
2. Do you experience bloating?
3. Do you frequently get hives?
4. Do you have an itchy scalp?
5. Do you have a white coating of the tongue?
6. Do you frequently get vaginal yeast infections?
7. Do you experience fatigue and brain fog after eating?
8. Do you have eczema?
9. Do you have a poor tolerance for alcohol?
10. Do you have irritable bowel syndrome?
11. Do you eat a high-carbohydrate diet?

For more in depth results please take our online self-assessment at: glutenfreeremedies.com

Scoring

Low Probability (less than 20%) 1-2 questions

Moderate Probability (50/50 chance) 3-4 questions

High Probability (over 75%) over 4 questions

Specific supplements may be helpful, based upon indicated symptoms:

1. If have a craving for sugar/sweets: Vegan Digestive Enzymes, Candidacillin, and Pau D'Arco

2. If you experience bloating: Candidacillin, Vegan Digestive Enzymes, and Triphala

3. If you frequently get hives: Candidacillin, Manjistha, and Eclipta Alba

4. If you have an itchy scalp: Candidacillin, Black Walnut Hulls, Eclipta Alba, and Manjistha

5. If you have a white coating of the tongue: Candidacillin

6. If you frequently get vaginal yeast infections: Leaky Gut Probiotic, Artemisia/Berberine, and Candidacillin

7. If you experience fatigue and brain fog after eating: Candidacillin, Acetyl L-Carnitine, and Leaky Gut Night

8. If you have eczema: Manjistha, Candidacillin, Black Walnut Hulls, and Eclipta Alba

9. If you have a poor tolerance for alcohol: Succinic Acid, Leaky Gut Aid Day, and Leaky Gut Aid Night

10. If you have irritable bowel syndrome: Leaky Gut Probiotic, Plant Digestive Enzymes, Vegan Digestive Enzymes, Mannan Oligosaccharides, and Triphala

Leaky Gut Syndrome

Leaky gut syndrome is a highly defined functional disorder of the gastrointestinal tract resulting from abnormal intestinal permeability. The intestinal mucosal membrane is inflamed, irritated, and compromised. Intestinal barrier dysfunction and damage to intestinal villi interfere with nutrient absorption, while permitting toxins, pathogens, and antigen–antibody complexes to enter the bloodstream. For further information about leaky gut, reference Chapter Seven.

Prolamine Intolerance

Gluten is a prolamine, a group of plant storage proteins that have high proline content. Prolamines are extremely resistant to degradation by the human digestive system. These storage proteins are found in seeds of cereal grains including wheat (gliadin), barley (hordein), rye (secalin), corn (zein), sorghum (kafirin), and oats (avenin). Prolamines are gluten type proteins and with the exception of kafirin, provoke inflammatory responses in susceptible individuals. Approximately 15–25% of patients with gluten intolerance and celiac disease are prolamine intolerant. These patients cannot safely eat corn or oats. A patient who is gluten free but develops symptoms upon consuming oats likely has a prolamine intolerance.

As an example of prolamine pathogenicity in susceptible individuals, avenin, oat-specific and avenin-reactive intestinal T cell lines have been isolated from patients with celiac disease. These T cell lines recognize avenin peptides complexed with HLA-DQ2. Avenins have amino acid sequences rich in proline that closely resemble wheat gluten antigenic peptide fragments (epitopes). Deamidation by tissue transglutaminase is involved in avenin epitope formation. Some celiac disease patients are susceptible to avenin-induced mucosal inflammation initiated by avenin-reactive intestinal mucosal T cells. Oat intolerance can cause intestinal pathology and symptoms in patients with celiac disease who are adhering to a strict gluten free diet, but are eating oats.

Cross-Reactivity

Foods that contain proteins similar in structure to prolamines are cross-reactive with gluten and provoke an analogous inflammatory response. These proinflammatory proteins include casein (contained in cow's milk), albumin (contained in chicken eggs), and soy protein. Regarding casein, dietary solutions include eliminating dairy products. In these cases goat and sheep milk, cheese, yogurt, and ice cream are usually well tolerated. Pure whey protein does not contain casein and is also acceptable. Regarding albumin, susceptible patients should eliminate foods containing chicken egg whites. The safety of chicken egg yolk remains controversial. Duck and quail eggs are safe to consume. Regarding soy protein, susceptible patients should eliminate soy containing foods from their diet. Soy based lecithin is usually well tolerated. Tamarind based sauce is a reasonable substitute for soy sauce. Approximately 60–70% of patients with gluten intolerance cross-react with casein, approximately 15–20% cross-react with egg white, and approximately 50% cross-react with soy.

Problematically, 70–80% of all gluten free products contain soy. Patients with gluten intolerance and celiac disease who are soy intolerant have to pay special attention to ingredient lists on such products. Vitamin E is also safe except for patients with a soy allergy.

Common Endocrine Abnormalities in Gluten Intolerant Individuals

As discussed in Chapter Four, people who are gluten tolerant can develop various abnormalities of the endocrine system, including:

- DHEA/DHEA sulfate deficiency
- Hashimoto's thyroiditis
- Hypothyroidism
- Insulin resistance
- Overproduction of prolactin
- Polycystic ovary disease
- Pregnenolone deficiency
- Testosterone deficiency

Diamine Oxidase Deficiency in Gluten Intolerant Individuals

Diamine oxidase deficiency is a common cause of elevated histamine levels in gluten intolerant individuals. When we eat, cells in the intestinal epithelial mucosa release histamine. Dilation of local blood vessels in response to histamine facilitates absorption of nutrients. At the appropriate time, the enzyme diamine oxidase breaks down histamine and absorption ceases, however diamine oxidase deficiency is found in gluten intolerance and celiac disease. In such clinical circumstances, histamine persists, causing prolonged vasodilation and leaky gut syndrome.

Histamine is a protein produced mainly by mast cells, platelets, and basophils. It is stored intracellularly in vesicles (small sacs) and released in the gastrointestinal tract in response to digestive processes and systemically in response to injury, inflammation, and allergic reactions. Histamine binding to target cell receptors causes contraction of smooth muscle, dilation of blood vessels, increased vascular permeability, mucus secretion, and arrhythmias. Many of these physiologic responses result in symptoms of allergies, including hives, sneezing, and a runny nose. Elevated histamine levels cause itching, upset stomach, and headaches. Overall, histamine causes inflammation as part of a local immune response.

The highest expression of diamine oxidase is in the small intestine, ascending portion of the large intestine, kidney, and placenta. Activity of diamine oxidase reflects the activity of the intestinal mucosa. For example, tissue diamine oxidase activity is diminished in inflammatory bowel disease and disorders like gluten intolerance and celiac disease that cause atrophy of intestinal mucosal structures. The balance between histamine and the histamine degrading enzyme, diamine oxidase, is crucial for achieving an uncomplicated pregnancy. Studies suggest that prolonged exposure of placental tissues to elevated levels of histamine can be implicated in the pathogenesis of pre-eclampsia (hypertension of pregnancy), intrauterine growth retardation, and spontaneous abortion, so gluten intolerance and celiac disease can be associated with numerous disorders of pregnancy.

Diamine oxidase deficiency is diagnosed by blood diamine oxidase level, blood histamine level, and blood N-methyl-histamine level. Its treatment is accomplished by supplementation with diamine oxidase obtained from porcine kidney and citrus-based bioflavonoids and bioflavonoids such as quercetin. These bioflavonoids stimulate production of diamine oxidase. Patients with diamine oxidase deficiency should maintain a histamine-free diet.

A strict histamine-free diet is a complicated protocol and involves avoiding the following foods:

- Fish
  - Anchovies
  - Mackerel
  - Sardines
  - Tuna
- Cheese
  - Camembert
  - Cheddar
  - Emmenthal
  - Gouda
  - Roquefort
  - Tilseter
- Meat
  - Dried ham
  - Hard-cured sausages
  - Salami
- Vegetables
  - Pickled cabbage
  - Spinach
  - Tomatoes (and ketchup)
- Alcoholic beverages
  - Beer
  - Red wine
  - Sparkling wine
  - White wine

Maintaining a strict gluten free diet is a necessary component in the treatment of gluten intolerance and celiac disease. If symptoms persist, additional triggers need to be investigated, identified, and addressed. Sources of potential gluten cross-contamination must also be identified and eliminated. Malabsorption associated nutrient deficiencies, prolamine intolerances, yeast infection in the gastrointestinal tract, leaky gut syndrome, endocrine disorders, and diamine oxidase deficiency can all play a role in perpetuating symptoms in patients with gluten intolerance and celiac disease. A rheumatologist or other specialist experienced in the treatment of gluten intolerance and celiac disease is needed to thoroughly investigate all potential sources of a patient's problems and will likely have a high index of clinical suspicion, the ability to engage in lateral thinking ("thinking outside the box"), and the determined relentlessness of a Sherlock Holmes as they engage in the process of solving a patient's challenging medical puzzles.

Basic Lifestyle Modifications When Living with Gluten Intolerance, Celiac Disease, and Related Conditions

For people with gluten intolerance and celiac disease, a strict gluten free diet for life is the first and most critical step in any comprehensive medical treatment plan needed to restore many patients to optimal good health, but some may have additional related disorders including leaky gut syndrome, yeast infection, prolamine intolerance, and/or diamine oxidase deficiency, and some may experience gluten cross-reactivity. Additional measures are necessary for these conditions. For all patients with gluten intolerance and celiac disease, learning the basics of initiating and maintaining a gluten free diet is the key to recovery. Understanding the principles of gluten cross-contamination and learning effective measures for avoiding these problems is the next step. Finally, learning how to recover from accidental gluten exposure provides tools that enable them to participate fully in day-to-day social and work-related activities. The knowledge gained provides patients with gluten intolerance and celiac disease with the ability to return to full, rich, and rewarding lives.

Basics of Gluten Free Living

For people with gluten intolerance and celiac disease, being on a gluten free diet is a lifelong requirement for good health.
It starts with elimination of foods containing the following grains:

- Barley
- Bulgur
- Durum
- Einkorn
- Farina
- Faro
- Graham
- Kamut
- Rye
- Semolina
- Spelt
- Triticale

It's important not start a gluten free diet "cold-turkey," as patients can experience gluten withdrawal symptoms like headaches, anxiety, agitation, abdominal discomfort, and nausea. They should allow 3 – 4 weeks to become gluten free and begin by eliminating major sources of gluten like bread, pasta, pizza, cake, cookies, and bagels, then eliminate minor sources of gluten. They need to be sure to obtain a gluten free toaster if someone else their home eats gluten containing bread.

Avoid the following food items and products unless they are labeled "gluten free:"

- Beer and ale
- Bread
- Bread mixes
- Brown rice syrup
- Cakes and pies
- Candies

- Cereals
- Communion wafers
- Cookies and crackers
- Croutons
- Dressings
- Drugs and over-the-counter medications
- Energy bars
- Flour and cereal products
- French fries
- Gravies
- Imitation bacon
- Imitation meat or seafood
- Lager
- Marinades
- Matzoh
- Nutritional supplements
- Pastas
- Processed luncheon meats
- Sauces, including soy sauce
- Seasoned rice mixes
- Seasoned snack foods such as potato and tortilla chips
- Self-basting poultry
- Soups and soup bases
- Stuffing
- Thickeners (roux)
- Vegetables in sauces

Patients may initially feel deprived by their diet's restrictions, but should try to stay positive and focus on the foods they can eat. Eventually, they'll realize that many products they miss (for example, bread, pizza, bagels, buns) are available in gluten free forms. Remember that all vegetables, fruits, nuts, most dairy products, unprocessed or non-marinated meats, fish, poultry, rice, and beans are naturally gluten free and healthy. It's important to make sure these foods are not processed or mixed with gluten containing grains, additives, or preservatives.

Many grains and starches are gluten free, including:

- Amaranth
- Arrowroot
- Brown rice
- Buckwheat
- Corn and cornmeal
- Flax
- Gluten-free flours (rice, soy, corn, potato, bean)
- Hominy (corn)
- Millet
- Montina
- Potato
- Quinoa
- Rice
- Sorghum
- Soy
- Sweet potato
- Tapioca
- Teff

Gluten free certified oats, when consumed in moderate amounts (no more than ¼ to ½ cup per day), are usually well tolerated by those with gluten intolerance and celiac disease.

Gluten Free Breakfast Ideas

- Cream of buckwheat
- Fried or scrambled eggs
- Fruits
- Gluten free bacon
- Gluten free bagels/muffins
- Gluten free cereals
- Gluten free waffles
- Yogurt and smoothies

Gluten Free Lunch and Dinner Ideas

- Gluten free corn tortillas
- Gluten free rice or risotto
- Meat, seafood, poultry
- Potato or sweet potato
- Rice noodle soup
- Sandwich on gluten free bread
- Steamed vegetables

Gluten Free Snack Ideas

- Air popped popcorn
- Cheese
- Dried fruits
- Fruits and vegetables
- Gluten free chips
- Gluten free crackers
- Nuts

Gluten Free Dessert Ideas

- Gluten free cakes/cookies/pie/cup cakes
- Gluten free ice cream
- Macaroons
- Meringue

Gluten Free Alcoholic Beverages

- Distilled alcoholic beverages
- Wine and hard liquor beverages
- Beer, ale, lager, and malt vinegars are not gluten free

Remember that non-food related sources of gluten can provoke symptoms of gluten intolerance and celiac disease. Non-food related sources of gluten include:

- After shave products
- Chewing gum
- Envelopes and postage stamp glue
- Hair dye
- Lipstick and lip balm
- Lotion
- Makeup
- Play-Doh
- Shampoo
- Soap
- Sunscreen and sunblock
- Toothpaste

Gluten Cross-Contamination

Cross-contamination occurs when gluten free foods come in contact with foods that contain gluten. Such cross-contamination can occur during the manufacturing process or at home if foods are prepared on common surfaces, or with utensils that weren't thoroughly cleaned after being used to prepare gluten containing foods. The following scenarios are common:

- Using a toaster for both gluten free bread and regular bread is a major source of cross-contamination
- Grills and barbecues, if not properly cleaned, may easily cross-contaminate foods. Many sauces used to barbecue contain gluten
- Mayonnaise, peanut butter, jam, and jelly jars are easily contaminated when making sandwiches
- Sifters used for both gluten containing and gluten free flours will cross-contaminate. At home, be sure to separate properly labeled sifters

Consider the steps needed to prevent cross-contamination at home, at school, and in the workplace.

Dr. Shikhman's Three Step Guide to Recover from Gluten Exposure

No matter how compliant a person is with their gluten free diet, they will experience accidental exposure to gluten, especially if they eat out or travel. Symptoms of gluten exposure vary depending on the amount of gluten consumed and their gluten reactivity threshold. Typically, small amounts of gluten trigger fatigue and brain fog lasting from several hours to several days. Consumption of moderate to large amounts triggers not only fatigue and brain fog, but also abdominal pain, diarrhea, headaches, joint pain, and stiffness. These symptoms can last from several days to several weeks. The following three action steps will help to recover from an episode of inadvertent gluten exposure by minimizing the unpleasant side effects.

Step One: Pre-Meal Preparation

The Gluten Breaker protocol will help avoid consequences associated with accidental gluten contamination. The procedure is to take two capsules immediately before and immediately after each meal. This approach is effective for accidental gluten contamination, but the protocol will not work for patients who knowingly consume gluten containing foods like pasta, breads, or cookies.

Gluten Breaker is a high-potency blend of plant derived enzymes specifically formulated to assist in degrading plant and animal proteins, including gluten, cow's milk casein, soy proteins, and lactose. The enzyme blend also hydrolyzes small peptides, including caseomorphins and gluteomorphins, which can adversely affect the central nervous system in susceptible individuals. Four capsules of Gluten Breaker can digest up to 1000mg of consumed gluten.

Step Two: Combat Exposure

If someone has already consumed gluten and are experiencing symptoms of exposure, take these actions:

- Start drinking plenty of fluids, preferably those with an alkaline pH. For example, dissolve ¼ teaspoon of baking soda in a glass of water and drink three to four glasses per day.
- Start taking Gluten Breaker, two capsules three times a day on an empty stomach (30 minutes before or 60 minutes after meals).
- Start taking N-Acetylglucosamine 2,000mg three times a day, and Mannan Oligosaccharides 2,000mg twice a day. Both supplements protect and regenerate the intestinal mucosal lining upon gluten exposure.
- Start taking Triphala, 500mg three times a day and 1,000–1,500mg before bedtime. Triphala is an ancient Ayurvedic herbal formula consisting of equal parts of three fruits (Harada, Amla, and Bihara). It is a laxative and colon cleanser. By increasing peristaltic movement of the intestine, Triphala accelerates removal of gluten residues from the digestive tract.

Step Three: Advanced Assistance

If there is no improvement after two or three days on Step Two, consider adding Yucca Schidigera Extract and GoldenBiotic-8. Yucca schidigera is a medicinal plant native to Mexico that contains several physiologically active phytochemicals like steroidal saponins that facilitate elimination of gluten from the digestive tract, stimulate growth of beneficial intestinal microorganisms, and relieve intestinal irritation. GoldenBiotic-8 is a proprietary blend of eight probiotic microorganisms specifically designed to restore gastrointestinal health in patients with malabsorption, leaky gut syndrome, and/or candidiasis. Certain probiotic strains in this formulation affect the GABA transmitting pathway and reduce symptoms of anxiety. In addition, these probiotics reduce intestinal inflammation and intestinal discomfort.

Conclusion

The strategies outlined in this chapter will get those with gluten intolerance on their way to feeling better by living a gluten free lifestyle. As they begin feeling better living gluten free, all of the things they thought they would miss will fade away as they begin to live a more healthy life. As always, patients need to follow up with all of their physician's recommendations and let their doctor know about any difficulties they encounter and any unusual or unexpected symptoms they may experience. Treatment of gluten intolerance and celiac disease is usually highly effective and their physician is their best resource to assist them in this life-long process.

In Conclusion

Learning you have gluten intolerance and celiac disease can be a major asset in returning to good health. This is true not only for those with gastrointestinal symptoms like diarrhea, constipation, abdominal pain, and abdominal swelling, but also for those with a variety of persistent, difficult to treat, and difficult to diagnose diseases and disorders.

Gluten intolerance and celiac disease are common conditions. Approximately 40% of the population has a genetic immunological signature that could predispose them to gluten intolerance, and approximately 1% of the U.S. population has celiac disease, which begins as gluten intolerance. In susceptible individuals, continued exposure to dietary gluten perpetuates the immune response and associated inflammatory reactions. The small intestine is the primary target tissue for the immune response and inflammation. With prolonged immune reactivity and inflammatory response, the small intestine develops characteristic changes in its inner lining that include damage and destruction of the tissues involved in digestion, causing the characteristic gastrointestinal symptoms of celiac disease.

During the past 25 years much research has been done on celiac disease, focusing on its causes, the spectrum of immunological involvement, and its broad range of related conditions. Medical researchers have learned that celiac disease is associated with autoimmune diseases like lupus, rheumatoid arthritis, and scleroderma, as well as endocrine diseases like type 1 diabetes, hyperthyroidism, hypothyroidism, Addison's disease, and fertility disorders. It is also associated with neuropsychiatric conditions including autism, attention deficit hyperactivity disorder, schizophrenia, seizure disorders, and malignancy. Discovering an association between celiac disease and difficult to treat conditions like autism or lupus may be the key to reducing the severity of symptoms and beginning a process of stabilization and/or recovery.

Gluten intolerance and celiac disease create great misery for affected people. The family physician refers them to an internist who refers them to a gastroenterologist, endocrinologist, neurologist, or psychiatrist. Blood is drawn and tests are performed. There may be additional referrals. Ultimately the diagnosis is unclear or inaccurate, so medications are prescribed that are not only ineffective, but cause additional problems. The patient becomes frustrated, discouraged, and may even become depressed. The patient suffers and the family suffers. There may be loss of income owing to the need to take personal and sick days. This downward spiral becomes self-perpetuating, as the nature of a critical underlying problem has not been identified. The primary obstacle to accurate diagnosis and institution of effective treatment is a lack of awareness of gluten intolerance and celiac disease.

Who needs to be evaluated for gluten intolerance and celiac disease? In answering this question, it's important to remember that celiac disease is a great mimicker. Its classical symptoms, abdominal pain, abdominal swelling, diarrhea, or constipation may be absent entirely. The only symptom of celiac disease might be an itchy, scaly skin eruption around the elbows, knees, scalp, and back (dermatitis herpetiformis). In such a case, an observant physician would consider celiac disease. If standard treatment for this class of skin lesions is not sufficiently effective, other diagnoses need to be considered. The bottom line is that any persistent symptoms involving the gastrointestinal, endocrine, immune, neurological, and dermatological systems requires further investigation, particularly to determine whether celiac disease is an underlying cause.

The immunological responses and inflammatory reactions of celiac disease may cause the development of other autoimmune diseases like lupus or rheumatoid arthritis, or participate in increasing the severity and quantity of symptoms of an autoimmune disease that is already present. The immunological and inflammatory nature of celiac disease may be the underlying or perpetuating cause of infertility, ADHD, or autism. Celiac disease can be a critical factor in the development of type 1 diabetes, schizophrenia, or fibromyalgia. In the optimal scenario, your physician will consider gluten intolerance and celiac disease as a potential factor, otherwise they must be considered whenever standard treatment for a serious condition is not achieving anticipated results.

Celiac disease is specifically diagnosed by laboratory tests that detect anti-tissue transglutaminase antibodies in a patient's blood, and by genetic testing that detects the presence of HLA DQ2 and/or HLA DQ8 immunological proteins. If celiac disease is diagnosed, the next step is to begin a three month trial of a strict gluten free diet. If symptoms improve during the gluten free trial, celiac disease is confirmed and the patient is placed on a gluten free diet for life.

In many patients symptoms improve quickly, often after one or two weeks on a gluten free diet. Neuropsychiatric symptoms and behaviors improve, and swelling and pain of autoimmune musculoskeletal diseases diminish and may begin to resolve. People with lifelong endocrine diseases affecting the pancreas, thyroid, or kidney improve, getting stronger and healthier as they clear their systems of gluten. Following a period of time on a gluten free diet, a woman who has been infertile or had several miscarriages may become pregnant and deliver a healthy baby. People with symptoms of fibromyalgia, sometimes for more than 10 years, begin to feel substantially better and are able to re-engage with their daily lives, making whole new worlds of possibility available.

The common thread in these diverse scenarios is the ability to identify and eliminate a specific contributing factor, gluten, which can cause non-gastrointestinal conditions like autism or infertility, or participate as an exacerbating mechanism in their development. Eliminating gluten enables valuable physiological resources to be directed toward healing associated problems rather than being diverted toward managing the effects of a related immunological and inflammatory disease — celiac disease. People with previously undiagnosed celiac disease who begin a gluten free diet for life report that they feel as if they've gotten their life back. Unmanageable symptoms become manageable, a good night's sleep becomes a common experience, and regular exercise becomes possible. People return to their normal weight, lifestyles improve, and they are able to think of themselves as healthy rather than sick.

The good news is that gluten intolerance and celiac disease are treatable. You don't have to live with unpleasant, stressful, and discouraging symptoms for the rest of your life. It's possible to control the effects of these disorders. The solution is to be on a gluten free diet for life. There is work involved in setting up and maintaining a gluten free diet, but the results make the effort worthwhile. Frequently the benefits are immediate, within the first few weeks of a gluten free diet, and the positive feedback assists in the process of reorganizing your kitchen. Many people report eating a healthier, more nutritious diet now that they're gluten free. Spouses and children of people with celiac disease often support their loved one by becoming gluten free themselves, making the new lifestyle a shared family experience.

Public awareness of gluten intolerance and celiac disease has increased in the last few years. Many local markets, health food stores, and supermarket chains now carry a wide selection of gluten free foods and household products. Gluten free items can also be easily purchased on the Internet. There are gluten free print magazines and Internet based gluten free blogs and journals. Physician awareness of gluten intolerance and celiac disease is necessary for timely diagnosis and treatment. Make sure your doctor is considering gluten intolerance and celiac disease if your symptoms are among those described in *The Glutened Human*.

Public awareness of gluten intolerance and celiac disease also impacts how family and friends interact with and support a child, teenager, or adult who has these conditions, which are lifelong disorders. An affected person is never "healed" in the sense that any exposure to gluten at any time will cause a return of symptoms. As gluten intolerance is an immunological reaction, exposure to it causes a cascading set of immunological and inflammatory responses. The person's health is affected as his or her body attempts to return to normal. Energy is expended as they cope with a sudden onset of symptoms and become sick with other disorders like autism, diabetes, arthritis, or fibromyalgia. Any exposure to gluten can have serious consequences.

When family and friends lack awareness of gluten intolerance and celiac disease, the affected person may feel unsupported and withdraw from the group. Well meaning people encourage them to "be like everyone else," offering foods the gluten intolerant person knows they should avoid. The family member or friend says, "Come on, you can eat a little bit, you'll be OK." That person is not aware of how injurious even a very small amount of gluten can be. FDA regulations state that gluten free food must have levels less than 20 parts per million, a small amount. The cupcake a well meaning adult offers to a gluten intolerant child at a birthday party contains far more gluten than 20 parts per million.

It is particularly important for children to have the experience of being taken care of. No child wants to be identified as "abnormal." A gluten intolerant child needs to be treated similarly to other children at gatherings, and their food requirements need to be handled seamlessly, without any sense of being "singled out."

The only cure for gluten intolerance and celiac disease is a strict gluten free diet for life, which means no gluten at any time, even at parties, holidays, and family functions. Family and friends can support gluten intolerant people including them in group activities centered around food, rather than by highlighting their dietary restrictions. If a host hasn't prepared any gluten free food, gluten free guests should be encouraged to bring their own food. Meal times and snack times can focus on camaraderie and friendship, making people free to celebrate their differences rather than being forced into a uniformity that will backfire by being deleterious to their health.

Some people find living a gluten free life too challenging. Finding joy in health, rather than in food, necessitates reframing one's perspective. Help your gluten intolerant loved ones by learning about this disorder and the dietary requirements. We are all subject to habit, especially when it comes to eating foods we truly like. Just as some people find that exercise is not fun until you begin to appreciate the benefits, the same is true of living gluten free. We can support each other in enjoying a life of greater vitality and health over the years.

When we focus on the big picture, we discover that effectively diagnosing and treating gluten intolerance and celiac disease significantly contributes not only to the patient's welfare and well being, but also to the welfare of society as a whole. Each of the diseases and disorders discussed in *The Glutened Human* is a lifetime condition. If going on a gluten free diet is appropriate for the specific condition, the result may be long term improvement, with long term benefits to that person, their family, and their community, both on a small and a large scale. A gluten free diet makes all the difference!

GLUTEN-FREE REMEDIES:

NATURAL SECRETS TO BETTER HEALTH

The importance of dietary supplements in treatment of celiac disease, gluten intolerance and associated diseases.

As a practicing physician and researcher, I realized early in my career that the successful treatment of chronic illnesses cannot completely rely on drugs—that an integrative approach including dietary modifications, food supplements and herbs can offer extraordinary results.

In addition, it became more and more obvious that gluten, a simple dietary grain protein, possesses an enormous 'virulent' potential and contributes to the development and progression of various chronic inflammatory and autoimmune diseases. Following a gluten-free diet can bring miraculous relief, but the elimination of gluten does not allow the body to get the critical nutrients it needs. The best way to compensate for lack of nutrients is to take dietary supplements. I wanted to provide a safe, worry-free option for the gluten intolerant community so I created Gluten-Free Remedies. Although conceptualized for those requiring a gluten free diet, they are suitable for everyone.

Launched in 2011, Gluten-Free Remedies combines our intimate knowledge of auto-immune disorders, gluten intolerance, nutrition, and holistic healing arts into a line of herbs and supplements of the utmost purity and quality. All of our products are certified gluten free by the Celiac Support Association and manufactured in facilities that follow the highest manufacturing standards. We continually develop new, proprietary products based on the latest research and proven solutions in the industry.

Our goal is to provide you a satisfying experience that will help you feel better, healthier, and happier.

Gluten-Free Remedies offers natural solutions for many chronic issues. Many of our supplements should be taken together to create a synergistic effect—often times protocols have multiple products that address various needs within a given symptom set.

There are a few protocols* that we have had great success with in our practice. This information is presented for educational purposes only and is not intended to replace the advice of your healthcare professional. Consult your doctor or health professional before starting a treatment or making any changes to your diet.

The products designated with a † are proprietary blends, exclusive to the Gluten-Free Remedies line that were formulated by Dr. Shikhman. You will not find these products anywhere else.

*These protocols have not been evaluated by the Food and Drug Administration. These are not intended to diagnose, treat, cure or prevent any disease.

Leaky Gut Syndrome

Product	Dosage (loading/severe symptoms)	Dosage (maintenance/light symptoms)
Leaky Gut Day†	2 caps in AM 2 caps at noon	1 cap in AM 1 cap at noon
Leaky Gut Night††	2 caps at night	1 cap at night
Leaky Gut Probiotic†	1-2 caps on an empty stomach	1 cap a day on an empty stomach
† proprietary blend exclusive to Gluten-Free Remedies		

Product	Ingredient Description
Leaky Gut Day	**Sodium Butyrate** controls intestinal permeability, modulates inflammation, suppresses yeast overgrowth, and optimizes intestinal motility. **Calcium D-Glucarate** inhibits glucuronidase, an enzyme that increases intestinal permeability, and facilitates the reabsorption of toxic substances through the intestinal wall.
Leaky Gut Night	**Calcium/Magnesium Butyrate** controls intestinal permeability, modulates inflammation, suppresses yeast overgrowth, and optimizes intestinal motility. **L-Glutamine** is an amino acid that plays a vital role in the maintenance of intestinal integrity and permeability.
Leaky Gut Probiotic	***Pediococcus acidilactici*** suppress growth of pathogenic bacteria. ***Lactobacillus plantarum*** feeds beneficial gut bacteria and kills pathogenic bacteria. ***Lactobacillus acidophilus*** supports good bacteria in the gut and prevents diarrhea.

Pain Management

Product	Dosage
RheumaNat†	1 cap twice a day (1000 mg)
Devil's Claw Plus†	1 cap twice a day (1500 mg)
Normogesic†	1 cap twice a day (1500 mg)
Butterbur/Feverfew Blend	1-2 caps twice a day (550 – 1100 mg)
Boswellia/Curcumin Blend	3 caps a day (1350 mg)
† proprietary blend exclusive to Gluten-Free Remedies	

Popular combinations:

Devils Claw Plus + RheumaNat + Normogesic: generalized pain, pain due to arthritis in hands, shoulders and knees, fibromyalgia, pain with insufficient response to pain killers.

Devil's Claw Plus+ Butterbur/Feverfew + Boswellia/Curcumin: generalized pain, neck and lower back pain.

Normogesic: pain due to inflammation.

Product	Ingredient Description
RheumaNat	**Iporuru Root Powder** controls muscle pain and joint pain, headaches as well as toothaches. The anti-inflammatory properties of iporuru are attributed to a group of alkaloids. Basic research demonstrates the anti-inflammatory activity of iporuru relies on its ability to inhibit cyclooxigenase (COX) enzymes responsible for mediating inflammation.
Devil's Claw Plus	**Devil's Claw Extract** possesses analgesic, anti-oxidant and anti-inflammatory activities. It inhibits various mediators of inflammation including COX-2, iNOS and suppresses translocation on nuclear factor kappaB (NF-kB). **Chuchuhuasi Bark Extract** used as a general remedy to relieve pain and inflammation, to treat arthritis, rheumatism and back pain.
Normogesic	**D-Phenylalanine** and **D-Leucine** enkephalin is a pentapeptide that regulates pain perception in the body. Enkephalinase is an enzyme which degrades enkephalins. Normogesic is a combination of two amino acids, D-phenylalanine and D-leucine, capable of blocking enkephalinase prolonging the life of enkephalins allowing for longer-lasting pain relief. L-Glutamine as a precursor neurotransmitter, L-Glutamine regulates pain perception in the brain. L-Tryptophane a precursor to neurotransmitter serotonin, which helps regulate pain.

Hair, Nail and Skin

Product	Dosage
Biotin	1-4 caps a day (5 – 20 mg)
Eclipta Alba	1-3 caps a day (500 – 1500 mg)
TruMarine Collagen	5 grams a day

Product	Ingredient Description
Biotin	**Biotin** is a key vitamin for maintaining integrity of hair and nails.
Eclipta Alba	**Eclipta Alba** promotes hair growth and reversal of graying hair.
TruMarine Collagen	**TruMarine Collagen** extracted from fish scales and skin, regularly improves skin moisture level, smoothness and suppleness. It prevents the signs of aging such as the formation of deep-winkles and fine lines as well as well as UVB-induced skin damage.

Osteoporosis

Product	Dosage
BoneDense†	1-3 caps twice a day (1000 – 3000 mg)
Strontium Citrate	2 caps a day (600 mg)
† proprietary blend exclusive to Gluten-Free Remedies	

Product	Ingredient Description
BoneDense	**Drynaria** inhibits osteoclast function and therefore decreases bone resorption and stimulates osteoblasts to produce more healthy bone tissue.
Strontium Citrate	**Strontium Citrate** is an element that is easily incorporated in the bones that improves low bone density.

Stress/Anxiety

Product	Dosage
Rhodiola	1-2 caps a day (500 – 1000 mg)
Eleutherococcus	2-4 caps a day (1000 – 2000 mg)

Product	Ingredient Description
Rhodiola	**Rhodiola** increases serotonin and dopamine-dependent processes in the central nervous system and stabilizes mood.
Eleutherococcus	**Eleutherococcus** an adaptogen which increases resistance to a variety of physical, chemical, or biological stressors.

Memory/Brain Fog

Product	Dosage
7 Keto	1-8 caps a day (25 – 200 mg)
Acetyl L Carnitine	2-6 caps a day (1000 – 3000 mg)
DMAE Plus†	2 caps twice a day (1200 mg)

Product	Ingredient Description
7 Keto	**7 Keto** supports memory and cognitive processes.
Acetyl L Carnitine	**Acetyl L Carnitine** a powerful brain booster and memory enhancer.

DMAE Plus†	**DMAE (dimethylaminoethanol)** is a chemical that is involved in a series of reactions that form acetylcholine, a chemical that is found in the brain and other areas of the body. Acetylcholine is a "neurotransmitter" that helps nerve cells communicate, decreases fatigue and improves attention. **L-Theanine** boosts alpha brain waves which lead to a feeling of relaxed and alert calmness and clarity. **Noopept** improved cognitive functions including improved clarity, better memory, and focus. **Piperine** increases nutrient absorption.
† proprietary blend exclusive to Gluten-Free Remedies	

Sleep

Product	Dosage
SAMe	The initial daily dose of varies from 1-6 caps a day (200 – 1200 mg) taken before bedtime for approximately 21 to 28 days. After that, the dosage can be reduced to maintenance levels of 1-2 caps a day (200 – 400 mg).
Sumenta	1-2 tablets a day
Taurine	1-3 caps a day (1000 – 3000 mg)

Product	Ingredient Description
SAMe	**SAMe** regulates synthesis of neurotransmitters (serotonin, melatonin, dopamine), hormones, homocysteine and glutathione.
Sumenta	**Key Ingredients:** **Ashwagndha** anxiolytic, neuroprotective, calms nervous system **Jatamansi** tranquilizing properties, neuroprotective **Tagar, Brahmi** induces sound sleep
Taurine	**Taurine** increases the number of GABA receptors in your brain. This helps boost levels of this brain chemical. Taurine calms neurons, or brain cells, helping you feel more relaxed.

Thyroid Support

Product	Dosage
Iodine	1 cap a day (325 mcg)
Myo-Inositol	1-3 caps a day (500 – 1500 mg)
Selenium	1 cap a day (200 mcg)

Product	Ingredient Description
Iodine	**Iodine** the thyroid gland actively absorbs iodide from the blood to make and release the T3 and T4 hormones into the blood. Significant iodine deficiency causes decreased thyroid function.
Myo-Inositol	**Myo-Inositol** thyroid function is controlled by the thyroid stimulating hormone (TSH). TSH mediates its function via inositol signaling pathways. Administration of Selenium and Myo-Inositol in people with Hashimoto's disease showed beneficial synergistic activity in the reduction of pathogenic autoantibodies and restoration of thyroid function.
Selenium	**Selenium** plays a key role in the function of the thyroid gland, by serving as a cofactor (or helper) for three of the four thyroid hormone deiodinases that convert T4 to T3 (the active hormone). Clinical and experimental data show that selenium may inhibit Hashimoto's disease and reduce autoantibodies (so-called anti-TPO antibodies) that attack the thyroid gland.

Candida (Yeast Overgrowth)

Product	Dosage
Candidacillin†	1 cap a day
Black Walnut Hulls/Pau D'Arco/Barberry†	2 caps twice a day (2000 mg)
† proprietary blend exclusive to Gluten-Free Remedies	

Product	Ingredient Description
Candidacillin	**Calcium Undecylenate** is an antifungal agent and inhibits conversion of yeast cells into the pathogenic form. **Calcium Disodium EDTA** has strong antifungal activities that help destroy negative microbial and fungal biofilms. **Caprylic Acid** possesses strong natural antimicrobial and antifungal activity, and inhibits growth of various microorganisms including Candida albicans. **Monolaurin** has strong antibacterial and other antifungal effects in vitro.
Black Walnut Hulls/Pau D'Arco/Barberry	**Black Walnut Hulls** contains natural tannins that kill parasites, yeast and fungus with antibiotic and antifungal effects. **Pau D' Arco** a powerful antifungal agent inhibiting the growth of Candida. **Barberry** eases inflammation due to candida infections.

Fatigue

Product	Dosage
Inosine	2 caps twice a day (2000 mg)
PABA	2 caps a day (1000 mg)
DMAE Plus†	2 caps twice a day (1200 mg)
Sulbutiamine Plus†	2 caps twice a day (1200 mg)
† proprietary blend exclusive to Gluten-Free Remedies	

Product	Dosage
Inosine	**Inosine** is a nucleoside which increases athletic performance, improves communication between neurons and induces interferon, a key molecule participating in body protection from viral infections.
PABA	**PABA** is para-aminobenzoic acid, a molecule which enhances production of folic acid by gut bacteria, induces interferon and reduces fatigue via anti-oxidative pathway.
DMAE Plus	**DMAE (dimethylaminoethanol)** is a chemical that is involved in a series of reactions that form acetylcholine, a chemical that is found in the brain and other areas of the body. Acetylcholine is a "neurotransmitter" that helps nerve cells communicate, decreases fatigue and improves attention.

	L-Theanine boosts alpha brain waves which lead to a feeling of relaxed and alert calmness and clarity. **Noopept** improved cognitive functions including improved clarity, better memory, and focus. **Piperine** increases nutrient absorption.
Sulbutiamine Plus	**Sulbutiamine** is a fat-soluble derivative of thiamine (vitamin B$_1$) that crosses the blood–brain barrier more readily than the actual thiamine and increases the levels of vitamin B1 in the brain. Sulbutiamine helps people who are dealing with chronic fatigue due to infectious processes. **Milk Thistle** keeps the liver functioning properly by preventing fat storage and uses fat as fuel. **Alpha Lipoic Acid** the body needs ALA to produce energy, because it plays a crucial role in mitochondria, the energy-producing structures in cells. **Piperine** increases nutrient absorption.

Dry Eyes and Mouth

Product	Dosage
SalivaStim†	2 caps a day in the am (1000 mg)
Black Currant Seed Oil	2-4 softgels a day (1000 – 2000 mg)
Krill Oil	2 softgels a day (1000 mg)
† proprietary blend exclusive to Gluten-Free Remedies	

Product	Ingredient Description
SalivaStim	**Dendrobium nobile** stimulates tear and saliva production by suppressing the inflammatory process in the salivary glands and restoring the expression and function of the the main water channel protein resulting in saliva production. **Smylax medica** improves perspiration benefitting mucosal and skin dryness.
Black Currant Seed Oil	**Black Currant Seed Oil** gamma-linolenic acid (GLA) decreases inflammation and prevents exacerbations.
Krill Oil	**Krill Oil** krill oil's unique combination of astaxanthin and phospholipid DHA is beneficial to eye health.

Subclinical adrenal insufficiency ("Adrenal fatigue")

Product	Dosage
Rhodiola	1-2 caps a day (500 – 1000 mg)
Eleutherococcus	2-4 caps a day (1000 – 2000 mg)
Pregnenolone	1-2 caps a day (25 – 50mg) WARNING: NOT FOR USE BY INDIVIDUALS UNDER THE AGE OF 18 YEARS. DO NOT USE IF PREGNANT OR NURSING.
7-Keto	1-8 caps a day (25 – 200 mg)
Licorice Root Extract	1 -3 caps a day (900 – 2700 mg)

Product	Ingredient Description
Rhodiola	**Rhodiola** increases serotonin and dopamine-dependent processes in the central nervous system and stabilizes mood.
Eleutherococcus	**Eleutherococcus** an adaptogen which increases resistance to a variety of physical, chemical, or biological stressors.
Pregnenolone	**Pregnenolone** possesses various biological effects including behaving as a neuroactive steroid and improves memory and cognitive function.
7-Keto	**7 Keto** has strong immune enhancing, memory enhancing and stress reducing action.
Licorice Root Extract	**Licorice Root** mimics the effects of cortisol which controls the release of energy in the body.

Inflammation management

Product	Dosage
Boswellia/Curcumin Blend	3 caps a day (1350 mg)
Curcupinol†	1 cap three times a day (2250 mg)
Devil's Claw Plus†	1 cap twice a day (1500 mg)
Pregnenolone	1-2 caps a day (25 – 50mg) WARNING: NOT FOR USE BY INDIVIDUALS UNDER THE AGE OF 18 YEARS. DO NOT USE IF PREGNANT OR NURSING.
RheumaNat†	1 cap twice a day (1000 mg)
† proprietary blend exclusive to Gluten-Free Remedies	

Product	Ingredient Description
Boswellia/Curcumin Blend	**Boswellic acid** expresses strong anti-inflammatory activity. **Curcumin** possesses a variety of biologic and pharmacologic activities, including anti-inflammatory, anti-oxidant, and anticarcinogenic ones.

Curcupinol	**Curcumin** shows strong anti-oxidation and anti-inflammatory activities.
	Pine Bark Extract contains over 95% of proanthocyanidins oligomeric flavonoids possessing strong anti-oxidant and anti-inflammatory activities. Proanthocyanidins have low acute and chronic toxicity and protect against oxidative stress in several cell systems by doubling the intracellular synthesis of anti-oxidative enzymes and by acting as a potent scavenger of free radicals.
	Oregon Grape Root Powder the main chemical constituents of Oregon grape root powder include berberine, berbamine, and oxyacanthine, both white alkaloids. Berberine has demonstrated significant antimicrobial activity against a variety of organisms.
	Piperine increases nutrient absorption.
Devil's Claw Plus	**Devil's Claw Extract** possesses analgesic, anti-oxidant and anti-inflammatory activities. It inhibits various mediators of inflammation including COX-2, iNOS and suppresses translocation on nuclear factor kappaB (NF-kB).
	Chuchuhuasi Bark Extract used as a general remedy to relieve pain and inflammation, to treat arthritis, rheumatism and back pain.

Pregnenolone	**Pregnenolone** possesses various biological effects including behaving as a neuroactive steroid and improves memory and cognitive function.
RheumaNat	**Iporuru Root Powder** controls muscle pain and joint pain, headaches as well as toothaches. The anti-inflammatory properties of iporuru are attributed to a group of alkaloids. Basic research demonstrates the anti-inflammatory activity of iporuru relies on its ability to inhibit cyclooxigenase (COX) enzymes responsible for mediating inflammation.

Probiotics

Product	Dosage
Leaky Gut Probiotic†	1-2 caps a day (75 – 150 billion Colony Forming Unit (CFU))
GoldenBiotic-8	1-4 caps a day (25 – 100 billion CFU)
Bacillus coagulans	1-3 caps a day (25 – 75 billion CFU)
Saccharomyces Boulardii	1 -4 caps a day (3 – 12 billion CFU)
† proprietary blend exclusive to Gluten-Free Remedies	

Product	Ingredient Description
Leaky Gut Probiotic	*Pediococcus acidilactici* suppress growth of pathogenic bacteria. *Lactobacillus plantarum* feeds beneficial gut bacteria and kills pathogenic bacteria. *Lactobacillus acidophilus* supports good bacteria in the gut and prevents diarrhea.
GoldenBiotic-8	**Most suitable for: general gut health, malabsorption, food intolerances.** *Lactobacillus acidophilus* the medicinal properties of L. acidophilus DDS-1 include: production of lactic acid supporting good bacteria in the gut, production of B and K vitamins, prevention of 'traveler's diarrhea', inhibition of gastric/duodenal ulcers caused by Helicobacter pylori, reduction of symptoms of eczema and atopic dermatitis, reduction of serum cholesterol level, fermentation of lactose and reduction of symptoms of lactose intolerance, reduction of intestinal pain.

Lactobacillus plantarum the medicinal properties of L. plantarum include: production of D- and L-isomers of lactic acid feeding beneficial gut bacteria, production of hydrogen peroxide killing pathogenic bacteria, production of enzymes (proteases) degrading soy protein and helping people with soy intolerance, synthesis of amino-acid L-lysine that promotes absorption of calcium and the building of muscle tissue, production of enzymes (proteases) digesting animal proteins such as gelatin and helping people with pancreatic insufficiency.

Lactobacillus casei the medicinal properties of L. casei include: production of lactic acid assisting propagation of desirable bacteria in the gut, fermentation of lactose and helping people with lactose intolerance.

Lactobacillus rhamnosus the medicinal properties of L. rhamnosus include: production of lactic acid supporting good bacteria in the gut, production of bacteriocins and hydrogen peroxide killing pathogenic bacteria, prevention of diarrhea, prevention of upper respiratory infections, reduction of symptoms of eczema and atopic dermatitis, affecting GABA neurotransmitting pathway and reducing symptoms of anxiety.

Lactobacillus salivarius the medicinal properties of L. salivarius include: production of lactic acid supporting good bacteria in the gut, reduction of inflammatory processes causing colitis and inflammatory arthritis.

Bifidobacterium bifidus the medicinal properties of B. bifidus include: production of hydrogen peroxide killing pathogenic bacteria, modulation of local immune responses, and production of vitamins B, K and folic acid.

Bifidobacterium lactis the medicinal properties of B. lactis include: production of hydrogen peroxide killing pathogenic bacteria, modulation of local immune responses, and production of vitamins B, K and folic acid.

Lactococcus lactis the medicinal properties of L. lactis include: production of lactic acid supporting good bacteria in the gut, fermentation of lactose and reduction of symptoms of lactose intolerance.

Bacillus coagulans	Most suitable for: various inflammatory conditions: rheumatoid arthritis, colitis, Crohn's disease, potentially – psoriasis, psoriatic arthritis, ankylosing spondylitis. Once in the intestines, Bacillus coagulans is activated and releases anti-inflammatory molecules or acts indirectly to eradicate organisms in the gut responsible for the inflammatory immune response.
Saccharomyces Boulardii	S. boulardii maintains and restores the natural flora in the large and small intestine. S. boulardii aids in the treatment and prevention of various gastrointestinal disorders.

Prebiotics

Prebiotics are non-digestible carbohydrate-based food ingredients that stimulate the growth of beneficial bacteria in the gastrointestinal tract. Prebiotics act as food for probiotics. You need a healthy amount of probiotics in your intestines to help keep your digestive system in balance. If you don't eat foods rich in prebiotics, your level of probiotics may fall.

Product	Dosage
Ultimate Prebiotic/ Galactooligosaccharides	6 grams a day
Mannan Oligosaccharides	The starting dose of MOS should be 500 mg 2 times a day. If this dose is tolerated, it can eventually escalate to 1000-3000 mg 2 times a day.

Product	Ingredient Description
Ultimate Prebiotic/ Galactooligosaccharides	**Most suitable for: Osteopenia and Osteoporosis, Irritable Bowel Syndrome, alleviates constipation, improves absorption of calcium and magnesium.** **Galactooligosaccharides** stimulates the growth of health-promoting bacteria such as Bifidobacteria and Lactobacilli and suppress the survival of pathogenic microorganisms. **Apple Pectin** is a gelling agent and impacts transit time, gastric emptying and nutrient absorption from the gut.

	Aloe Vera Gel possesses purgative properties. **Licorice Root** has antiviral, anti-inflammatory, anti-tumor, and antimicrobial properties. Possesses gastroprotective activity and normalizes intestinal permeability.
Mannan Oligosaccharides	**Most suitable for: chronic yeast and gastrointestinal infections, celiac disease, and damaged small intestine.** **Mannan Oligosaccharides** stimulate the growth of beneficial microorganisms in the intestinal lumen and optimize immune responses. MOS detaches bad bacteria from the intestinal wall, restores intestinal villi and stimulates digestive enzymes.

Dr. Shikhman's Three Step Guide to Recover from Gluten Exposure

No matter how compliant a person is with their gluten free diet, they will experience accidental exposure to gluten, especially if they eat out or travel. Symptoms of gluten exposure vary depending on the amount of gluten consumed and their gluten reactivity threshold. Typically, small amounts of gluten trigger fatigue and brain fog lasting from several hours to several days. Consumption of moderate to large amounts triggers not only fatigue and brain fog, but also abdominal pain, diarrhea, headaches, joint pain, and stiffness. These symptoms can last from several days to several weeks. The following three action steps will help to recover from an episode of inadvertent gluten exposure by minimizing the unpleasant side effects.

Step One: Pre-Meal Preparation

The Gluten Breaker protocol will help avoid consequences associated with accidental gluten contamination. The procedure is to take two capsules immediately before and immediately after each meal. This approach is effective for accidental gluten contamination, but the protocol will not work for patients who knowingly consume gluten containing foods like pasta, breads, or cookies.

Gluten Breaker is a high-potency blend of plant derived enzymes specifically formulated to assist in degrading plant and animal proteins, including gluten, cow's milk casein, soy proteins, and lactose. The enzyme blend also hydrolyzes small peptides, including caseomorphins and gluteomorphins, which can adversely affect the central nervous system in susceptible individuals. Four capsules of Gluten Breaker can digest up to 1000mg of consumed gluten.

Step Two: Combat Exposure

If someone has already consumed gluten and are experiencing symptoms of exposure, take these actions:

- Start drinking plenty of fluids, preferably those with an alkaline pH. For example, dissolve ¼ teaspoon of baking soda in a glass of water and drink three to four glasses per day.
- Start taking Gluten Breaker, two capsules three times a day on an empty stomach (30 minutes before or 60 minutes after meals).
- Start taking N-Acetylglucosamine 2,000mg three times a day, and Mannan Oligosaccharides 2,000mg twice a day. Both supplements protect and regenerate the intestinal mucosal lining upon gluten exposure.
- Start taking Triphala, 500mg three times a day and 1,000–1,500mg before bedtime. Triphala is an ancient Ayurvedic herbal formula consisting of equal parts of three fruits (Harada, Amla, and Bihara). It is a laxative and colon cleanser. By increasing peristaltic movement of the intestine, Triphala accelerates removal of gluten residues from the digestive tract.

Step Three: Advanced Assistance

If there is no improvement after two or three days on Step Two, consider adding Yucca Schidigera Extract and GoldenBiotic-8. Yucca schidigera is a medicinal plant native to Mexico that contains several physiologically active phytochemicals like steroidal saponins that facilitate elimination of gluten from the digestive tract, stimulate growth of beneficial intestinal microorganisms, and relieve intestinal irritation. GoldenBiotic-8 is a proprietary blend of eight probiotic microorganisms specifically designed to restore gastrointestinal health in patients with malabsorption, leaky gut syndrome, and/or candidiasis. Certain probiotic strains in this formulation affect the GABA transmitting pathway and reduce symptoms of anxiety. In addition, these probiotics reduce intestinal inflammation and intestinal discomfort.

Bibliography

Aldana S: The Culprit and the Cure. Mapleton, UT, Maple Mountain Press, 2005

Askling J, et al: Cancer incidence in a population-based cohort of individuals hospitalized with celiac disease or dermatitis herpetiformis. Gastroenterology 123(5):1428-1435, 2002

Atladottir HO, et al: Association of family history of autoimmune diseases and autism spectrum disorder. Pediatrics 124(2):687-694, 2009

Autism and Developmental Disabilities Monitoring Network. Atlanta, GA, Centers for Disease Control and Prevention, 2007

Berg L, et al: Interferon-gamma production in response to in vitro stimulation with collagen type II in rheumatoid arthritis is associated with HLA-DRB1 and HLA-DQ8. Arthritis Res 2(1):75-84, 2000

Berti I, et al: Usefulness of screening program for celiac disease in autoimmune thyroiditis. Dig Dis Sci 45(2):403-406, 2000

Bethune MT, Khosla C: Parallels between pathogens and gluten peptides in celiac sprue. PLOS Pathogens 4(2):1-16, 2008 (e34)

Brown RT, et al: Prevalence and assessment of attention-deficit/hyperactivity disorder in primary care settings. Pediatrics 107(3):E43, 2001

Bushara KO: Neurologic presentation of celiac disease. Gastroenterology 128(4 Suppl 1):S92-S97, 2005

Cade R, et al: Autism and schizophrenia. Intestinal disorders. Nutritional Neurosci 3(1):57-72, 2000

Catassi C, et al: Celiac disease in the general population. Should we treat asymptomatic cases? J Pediatr Gastroenterol Nutr 24(Suppl 1):10-13, 1997

Catassi C, et al: Risk of non-Hodgkin's lymphoma in celiac disease. JAMA 287(11):1413-1419, 2002

Centers for Disease Control and Prevention: 10 Things to Know About New Autism Data— http://www.cdc.gov/features/dsautismdata/index.html

Centers for Disease Control and Prevention: Key Findings: Trends in the Parent-Report of Health Care Provider-Diagnosis and Medication Treatment for ADHD: United States, 2003—2011— http://www.cdc.gov/ncbddd/adhd/features/key-findings-adhd72013.html

Ch'ng CL, et al: Prospective screening for coeliac disease in patients with Graves' hyperthyroidism using anti-gliadin and tissue transglutaminase antibodies. Clin Endocrinol 62(3):303-306, 2005

Counsell CE, et al: Coeliac disease and autoimmune thyroid disease. Gut 35:844-846, 1994

Cuoco L, et al: Prevalence and early diagnosis of coeliac disease in autoimmune thyroid disorders. Ital J Gastroenterol Hepatol 31(4):287-287, 1999

da Rosa Utiyama SR, et al: Spectrum of autoantibodies in celiac patients and relatives. Dig Dis Sci 46(12):2624-2630, 2001

Diet and Behavior in Young Children with Autism—Clinical Trials Registry—http://clinicaltrials.gov/ct2/show/NCT00090428

Dietary Intervention in Autism—Clinical Trials Registry— http://clinicaltrials.gov/ct2/show/NCT00614198

Dieterich W, et al: Identification of tissue transglutaminase as the autoantigen of celiac disease. Nature Med 3(7):797-801, 1997

Dohan FC: Wheat consumption and hospital admissions for schizophrenia during World War II. A preliminary report. Am J Clin Nutr 18:7-10, 1966

Duntas LH: Does celiac disease trigger autoimmune thyroiditis? Nat Rev Endocrinol 5(4):190-191, 2009

Elder JH, et al: The gluten-free, casein-free diet in autism. Results of a preliminary double-blind clinical trial. J Autism Dev Dis Disord 36(3):413-420, 2006

Fasano A: Systemic autoimmune disorders in celiac disease. Clin Opin Gastroenterol 22(6):674-679, 2006

Firestein GS: Evolving concepts of rheumatoid arthritis. Nature 423:356-361, 2003

Fracchia M et al: Co-occurrence of celiac disease and other autoimmune diseases in celiacs and their first-degree relatives. Dig Liver Dis 36(7):489-491, 2004

Freeman HJ: Adult celiac disease followed by onset of systemic lupus erythematosus. J Clin Gastroenterol 42(3):252-255, 2008

Gough KR, et al: Intestinal reticulosis as a complication of idiopathic steatorrhoea. Gut 3:232-239, 1962

Graff H, Handford A: Celiac syndrome in the case histories of four schizophrenics. Psychiatr Q 35:306-313, 1961

Green PHR, Cellier C: Celiac disease. N Engl J Med 357(17):1731-1743, 2007

Green PHR, et al: Risk of malignancy in patients with celiac disease. Am J Med 115:191-195, 2003

Hadjivassiliou M, et al: Gluten ataxia. Cerebellum 7(3):497-498, 2008

Hadjivassiliou M, et al: Gluten sensitivity. Exploring the neurological iceberg. In Abstracts of the Seventh International Symposium on Coeliac Disease. Tampere, Finland, Vammalan Kirjapaino, 1996, 41(a)

Health, United States, 2008. Atlanta, GA, Centers for Disease Control and Prevention, Table 26. http://www.cdc.gov/nchs/fastats/lifexpec.htm

Holmes GKT, et al: Malignancy in coeliac disease. Effect of a gluten-free diet. Gut 30:333-338, 1989

Jyonouchi H, et al: Innate immunity associated with inflammatory responses and cytokine production against common dietary proteins in patients with autism spectrum disorder. Neuropsychobiology 46:76-84, 2002

Kagnoff MF: Celiac disease. Pathogenesis of a model immunogenetic disease. J Clin Invest 117(1):41–48, 2007

Kalaydjian AE, et al: The gluten connection. The association between schizophrenia and celiac disease. Acta Psychiatr Scand 113:82-90, 2006

Koning F, et al: Gluten: a two-edged sword. Immunopathogenesis of celiac disease. Springer Semin Immunol 27:217-232, 2005

Lepore L, et al: Prevalence of celiac disease in patients with juvenile chornic arthritis. J Pediatr 129:311-313, 1996

Lerner A, et al: Increased prevalence of autoantibodies in celiac disease. Dig Dis Sci 43(4):723-726, 1998

Lewis CM, et al: Genome scan meta-analysis of schizophrenia and bipolar disorder. Part II. Schizophrenia. Am J Hum Genet 73:34-48, 2003

Lidén M, et al: Gluten sensitivity in patients with primary Sjögren's syndrome. Scand J Gastroenterol 42(8):962-967, 2007

Loftus CG, Loftus EV Jr: Cancer risk in celiac disease. Gastroenterology 123(5):1726-1729, 2002

Lohi S, et al: Malignancies in cases with screening-identified evidence of coeliac disease. A long-term population-based cohort study. Gut 58:643-647, 2009

Ludvigsson JF, et al: A Nationwide Study of the Association Between Celiac Disease and the Risk of Autistic Spectrum Disorders. JAMA Psychiatry 70(11):1224-1230, 2013

Marai I, et al: IgA and IgG tissue transglutaminase antibodies in systemic lupus erythematosus. Lupus 13:241-244, 2004

Marsh MN: Transglutaminase, gluten and celiac disease. Food for thought. Nature Med 3(7):725-726, 1997

Midhagen G, et al: Adult celiac disease within a defined geographic area in Sweden. Scan J Gastroenterol 23:1000-1004, 1988

Millward C, et al: Gluten- and casein-free diets for autistic spectrum disorder. Cochrane Database Syst Rev 16(2):CD003498), 2004

Millward C, et al: Gluten- and casein-free diets for autistic spectrum disorder. Cochrane Database Syst Rev Apr 16(2):CD003498, 2008 [update]

Mirza N, et al: Celiac disease in a patient with systemic lupus erythematosus: a case report and review of literature. Clin Rheumatol 26(5):827-828, 2007

Mohammed I, et al: Multiple immune complexes and hypocomplementaemia in dermatitis herpetiformis and celiac disease. Lancet II:487-490, 1976

Molberg Ø, Sollid LM: A gut feeling for joint inflammation. Using celiac disease to understand rheumatoid arthritis. Trends Immunol 27(4):188-194, 2006

Mukamel M, et al: Celiac disease associated with systemic lupus erythematosus. Isr J Med Sci 30:656-658, 1994

Nabozny GH, et al: HLA-DQ8 transgenic mice are highly susceptible to collagen-induced arthritis. J Exp Med 183(1):27-37, 1996

Naiver AJ, et al: Tissue transglutaminase antibodies in individuals with celiac disease bind to thyroid follicles and extracellular matrix and may contribute to thyroid dysfunction. Thyroid 18(11):1171-1172, 2008

National Institute of Mental Health: What is Attention Deficit Hyperactivity Disorder?
http://www.nimh.nih.gov/health/topics/attention-deficit-hyperactivity-disorder-adhd/index.shtml

National Institutes of Health Consensus Statement on Celiac Disease. NIH Consensus and State-of-the-Art Statements 21:1, 2004

Nelson DA: Gluten-sensitive enteropathy (celiac disease). More common than you think. Am Fam Phys 66(12):2259-2266, 2002

Neuhausen RL et al: Co-occurrence of celiac disease and other autoimmune diseases in celiacs and their first-degree relatives. J Autoimmun 31(2):160-165, 2008

Niederhofer H, Pittschieler K: A preliminary investigation of ADHD symptoms in persons with celiac disease. J Atten Disord 10(2):200-204, 2006

Parke AL, et al: Coeliac disease and rheumatoid arthritis. Ann Rheum Dis 43:378-380, 1984

Pelsser LM, Buitelaar JK: Favourable effect of a standard elimination diet on the behavior of young children with ADHD. A pilot study. Ned Tijdschr Geneeskd 146(52):2543-2547, 2002

Pelsser LM, et al: A randomised controlled trial into the effects of food on ADHD. Eur Child Adolesc Psychiatry 18(1):12-19, 2009

Schuppan D, Junker Y: Turning swords into plowshares. Transglutaminases to detoxify gluten. Gastroenterology 133(3):1025-1028, 2007

Schuppan D: Current concepts of celiac disease pathogenesis. Gastroenterology 119(1):234-242, 2000

Silano M, et al: Delayed diagnosis of coeliac disease increases cancer risk. BMC Gastroenterol 7:8, 2007

Silano M, et al: Effect of a gluten-free diet on the risk of enteropathy-associated T-cell lymphoma in celiac disease. Dig Dis Sci 53:972-976, 2008

Straub RE, et al: A potential vulnerability locus for schizophrenia on chromosome 6p24-22. Nat Genet 11:287-293, 1995

Teppo AM, Maury CP: Antibodies to gliadin, gluten and reticulin glycoprotein in rheumatic disease. Elevated levels in Sjögren's syndrome. Clin Exp Immunol 57(1):73-78, 1984

Valicenti-McDermott MD, et al: Gastrointestinal symptoms in children with an autism spectrum disorder and language regression. Pediatr Neurol 39(6):392-398, 2008

Varkel Y, et al: Simultaneous occurrence of systemis lupus erythematosus and coeliac disease-like features. Postgrad Med J 65:600-602, 1989

Ventura A, et al: Duration of exposure to gluten and risk of autoimmune disorders in patients with celiac disease. Gastroenterology 117:297-303, 1999

Ventura A: Coeliac disease and autoimmunity. In Lohiniemi S, et al: Changing Features of Coeliac Disease. Tampere, The Finnish Coeliac Society, 1998, pp 67-72

Walker WA, Isselbacher KJ: Uptake and transport of macromolecules by the intestine. Possible role in clinical disorders. Gastroenterology 67:531-550, 1974

Wei J, Hemmings GP: Gene, gut, and schizophrenia. The meeting point for the gene-environment interaction in developing schizophrenia. Med Hypotheses 64:547-552, 2005

West J, et al: Malignancy and mortality in people with coeliac disease. Population-based cohort study. BMJ 329(7468):716-719, 2004

Wills S, et al: Autoantibodies in autism spectrum disorder. Ann NY Acad Sci 1107:79-91, 2007

Wilson JM: The evaluation of the worth of early disease detection. J R Coll Gen Pract 16(Suppl 2):48-57, 1968

http://apps.fas.usda.gov/psdonline/circulars/production.pdf World Agriculture Production Circular Series WAP 2 16 February 2016

Young J: Common co-morbidities seen in adolescents with attention deficit hyperactivity disorder. Adolesc Med State Art Rev 19(2):216-228, 2008

Zelnick N, et al: Range of neurologic disorders in patients with celiac disease. Pediatrics 113(6):1672-1676, 2004

Zhong F, et al: An autosomal screen for genes that predispose to celiac disease in the western counties of Ireland. Nat Genet 114:329-333, 1996

ABOUT THE AUTHORS

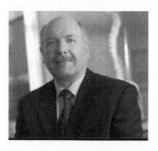

Board certified in internal medicine and rheumatology, Dr. Shikhman received his MD Cum Laude from the Russian State Medical University and his Ph.D. in Immunology from the Moscow Medical Academy. He served his internship and residency in internal medicine at the Oklahoma University Health Sciences Center and completed his clinical fellowship in rheumatology at Scripps Clinic. Subsequently, he became a member of Scripps Clinic Division of Rheumatology and a faculty member in the Department of Arthritis Research at the Scripps Research Institute. Additional training includes: medical acupuncture at UCLA, master classes in musculoskeletal ultrasound, auricolotherapy and auriculodiagnosis, and application of low-level lasers in therapy of arthritis and allied conditions.

He founded Institute for Specialized Medicine in 2008 as the nation's first clinic of integrative rheumatology. The clinic offers a holistic approach to healthcare; one that evaluates the total body to get to the root of the problem. Specializing in arthritis and autoimmune diseases, IFSMED brings diagnosis and care together offering all-inclusive service in one location. Gluten-free himself, he specializes in the connection between gluten and autoimmune diseases. In 2011, he launched a line of all natural gluten free supplements, Gluten-Free Remedies™, which help treat the complications that can arise from celiac disease.

www.ifsmed.com

www.glutenfreeremedies.com

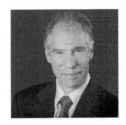

David Lemberg, M.S., D.C., received his M.S. in Bioethics from the Alden March Bioethics Institute at Albany Medical College. Dr. Lemberg is the author of *Taking Care at the End of Life: Five Steps to Writing a Meaningful and Practical Advance Directive.* His research interests include the intersection between science and society, health care policy, and environmental sustainability. Dr. Lemberg was the Executive Producer of SCIENCE AND SOCIETY, an Internet radio program presenting original content (2003-2012). He has interviewed more than 600 world leaders in the fields of biomedical research, genetics and genomics, health care policy, energy policy, nanotechnology, and science education.

ACKNOWLEDGEMENTS

To Kate Kurt, a quiet angel of Institute for Specialized Medicine and Gluten-Free Remedies, who made the publication of this book happen.

To Cherie Kephart for sharing your story and excellent editorial skills.

To Matt Pallamary for your editing expertise and guidance through the publication process.

To Marshall Ross for a superb help with cover design.

To my wife Galina who has supported my endeavors for over 35 years.

To all patients of Institute for Specialized Medicine and customers of Gluten-Free Remedies who intellectually stimulate our journey into the amazing world of medicine and integrative health.

All the patient's stories in this book are real. The actual names of patients were modified to protect their privacy.

46587174R00171

Made in the USA
San Bernardino, CA
10 March 2017